# Project You

# Reclaim Your Body With My 'No Diet' Formula

Lisa Ali

Copyright © 2018 Lisa Ali

All rights reserved.

ISBN-13: 9781796364859

# DEDICATION

For my beloved Mum, Sheelagh, who always believed in me, and who I think would be really proud!

# CONTENTS

|   | Acknowledgments | i |
|---|---|---|
| 1 | Introduction | 1 |
| 2 | Diet | 7 |
| 3 | Exercise | 33 |
| 4 | Lifestyle | 44 |
| 5 | Stress & Overwhelm | 61 |
| 6 | Motivation | 69 |
| 7 | Habits & Routines | 80 |
| 8 | Conclusion | 92 |
| 9 | Next Steps | 97 |

## ACKNOWLEDGMENTS

Thanks to all my lovely clients who have taught me so much, some of whom feature in here. Without them I wouldn't learn, grow and be able to help more people.

And to my husband, Terry. If it wasn't for him, his love, support and endless patience, I wouldn't have started this journey.

# 1 INTRODUCTION

"You've ballooned in front of my eyes. You can't tell me what to do".

Ouch!

After two and a half years away, I'd gone back into contract work. I was living half the week in a hotel in London, and the other half at home. To sum it up: I was miserable. Within the first month of being there, I'd booked a holiday to the USA as something to look forward to. A little glimmer of positivity.

Very quickly I was ten pounds, and soon fifteen pounds heavier. By the time I got back from the States I was over twenty pounds heavier than when I began that job. The pressure of delivering on the new contract was intense. The hours were long. When I finished work I'd go straight into the hotel bar and order a large glass of wine, carry on working at the bar for an hour or two, while I had another large glass of wine. Then it'd be 9pm and I would remember I still need to go out and get some food. Usually I couldn't be bothered, so I'd just eat whatever I could get at the hotel. This was typically a burger and chips, or something similar.

I hated the contract. I'd say it was the worst contract I've ever had. Even more than the work, I hated how I was letting myself go. Before going back into contract work I had been working as a Personal Trainer, teaching fitness classes. Now I was twenty pounds heavier just a couple of months later. I kept thinking to myself, "you know what to do, just do it". I knew I was drinking too much and eating rubbish. I knew I should do a bit of exercise in the hotel room. The problem was, I just couldn't bring myself to do it.

I sat down one day and had a very frank conversation with my husband. He said, "you've ballooned in front of my eyes". He went on to say, "you can't tell me what to do, you don't practice what you preach".

That was a tough conversation. I cried— not because what he said was mean— because it was true. My husband is not a cruel man, but he can be blunt. They say that the truth hurts, and I can attest it bloody hurt. When I stopped to think about it, I knew he was dead right.

This was the trigger for me to start looking to make changes in my life. The plan of going back into contract work was always supposed to be a temporary thing. I wanted to get back into health and fitness, I just didn't know how that would be yet. I guess you could say I ended up where I am now after an interesting journey, but more on that later.

I'd seen this Body Transformation Coach called Tim online. We were friends on Facebook. He put a post out one day saying he was looking to help women entrepreneurs who wanted to lose weight. I wasn't exactly an entrepreneur, but I reached out to him anyway and we had a conversation about what I needed to do.

I realised that I needed help. My husband was right— how could I help other people when I was overweight and unfit myself? I was overeating and drinking too much, I needed some help myself before I thought about trying to help other people.

Talking to Tim I told him that I wanted to lose about one-and-a-half stone. He said, "oh, about twenty pounds". That hit me like a ton of bricks. It wasn't just ten pounds or less. That double figure number seemed much further away. It wasn't a few pounds that I could lose quickly. It dawned on me just how far I had slipped, and the mountain I had to climb to get back to where I was.

Immediately I hired Tim and we started working together. I could easily have put it off, I could have made an excuse, but this time I didn't. It was about three weeks before the anniversary of my mum's passing. I'd gone back into work as an interim— at least partly— because I was so knocked off course by her death that I didn't know which way was up. Going back to something I knew was the easy option. The time around the anniversary was a difficult period for me, but I started the coaching anyway.

I was basically in free fall the week before and after the anniversary. Eating and drinking too much again. My weight had spiked back up, and I had to have a conversation with myself. I'd invested in myself, getting Tim's help, and I had to ask whether I wanted to do this or not.

We talked a lot about my mum and the struggles I was having. He would ask, "what can you do this week?". Instead of telling me to get over it and do more, he was asking if I could do one exercise session this week? He made it ok to give myself a break, to not worry and not beat myself up if I felt I hadn't done enough or had not been perfect.

I imagined what my mum would say. She'd have said, "Don't do it on my account darling. Don't use me as an excuse to hurt yourself". That was meaningful for me. I'd invested in making this transformation and I knew she would want me to be living a healthier, happier life. Tim showed me the power of coaching and the idea of finding the things that would help me move forward, instead of what is 'perfect', but wouldn't be realistic to follow.

The truth is, my transformation was simple. However, it wasn't easy due to my personal trauma and the demands of my job as an interim. Ultimately it came down to a choice; to just do it. There was a point where I realised the decision was mine, whether I wanted to change this part of my life or not was up to me. Once I'd had that conversation with myself, I knew I could make a whole heap of excuses to let myself off the hook, but I didn't. After that I just knuckled down and did it. I made the fundamental decision that I *was* doing this.

Having made that decision, it became easy. I was doing exercise in the tiniest space in my hotel room, but it didn't matter. I was finding a way to get it done, not because my situation was different or better, but because I committed to myself that this is what I am doing.

Soon after that I moved to my friend's house, which was a longer journey to work, but I couldn't bare living in a Travel Lodge any longer. When I started staying there I was taking better care of my food. Making better choices around what I ate because I had a kitchen again.

It was a lightbulb moment when I realised that I could be in control. By the end of the twelve weeks working with Tim I'd lost twenty pounds. I was back where I wanted to be, but it made me realise that this was still settling. That I could go further. I wasn't overweight, I was at that 'OK' place. A size twelve fit nicely and that was good, but I knew I could do more. In the coming months I went on to lose another twenty-five pounds. I did a photoshoot at my lightest, as the end of my weight loss journey, and now I'm settled somewhere comfortable in between the two.

When I did the photoshoot size eight clothes were falling off me. I never imagined I could have got back to that size, until I did it. I hadn't been that size since my early twenties. It was as though I was a different person. My confidence and belief had completely transformed. Taking this new-found belief in myself, I left the job that I hated and this time it was for good.

I started my fitness coaching part-time originally, while I was preparing for my photoshoot, with the view to build up the business and eventually go full-time. The manager of the contract I was on had said that they were getting rid of all the interims in September. I had a holiday in August anyway. The timing was perfect, and it just felt right. I decided I wasn't going to go back— it was time to bite the bullet and go into full-time coaching.

It was the perfect opportunity. I didn't want to be an interim any more, I didn't want to be in London any more. Having done my own transformation, I was now so confident in fitness, and my ability to help other people who have struggled with their own weight loss. I've never looked back since…

## Who Is This Book For?

This book is for anyone who has ever tried a diet and not got the results they had hoped. Anyone who is sick of starting the latest new diet. Anyone who's ever struggled with their weight and is worried that this is how they are going to be for the rest of their life. Anyone who is settling because they don't believe it's possible to change and achieve the results they really want.

It's for women and men who are busy, are competent in their work life and family life; but struggle to put themselves first and often find themselves bottom of their long list of priorities. It works well for people who have to travel for work; living half the week away from home in a hotel. This is the programme that I went through myself when I was a professional career interim. This gives me a unique understanding of what the day-to-day life is like, and the challenges that you often face when you're working contracts.

Treating yourself as a project, "Project You", is like taking a job. You don't focus on the outcome. You focus on the inputs and know that the outcome will take of itself. You have a project plan that you put together and follow. This book is the project plan for your health and body.

It is a sustainable plan, rather than the latest quick fix. If you know that if you don't do something about this now, nothing will ever change, then this is for you. It's for people who look in the mirror and refuse to continue thinking "well this is what forty— going in to old age— looks like". People who have decided that when they look in the mirror, they can see a different person looking back. It doesn't have to remain the way it is right now. There is a different way; a better way.

In project planning you have the project triangle of time, cost, and quality. All three need to align for a successful project. If you don't have the right budget, the right timeline in place; you're not going to be able to deliver on the plan. If the quality isn't up to scratch, it's meaningless anyway. This book will align those pieces for your body transformation through nutrition, exercise, lifestyle, mindset and creating sustainable habits.

If your project plan requires three times the budget you have, it is simply not going to work— you cannot do it. If your fitness plan requires you going to the gym five times a week, when you hate the gym, it is simply not going to work— you cannot do it. When I started applying project thinking to personal transformation, I was able to come up with my *Project You* methodology that works, is repeatable, and consistently gets great results for myself and my clients.

## What To Expect

This book is practical, simple, and effective. You might think that things can't be this simple and work, but they can. Follow the steps laid out, go through the process.

Focus on the task at hand; if you can break these tasks down like you would a project plan, you will get the outcome you're looking for. You simply have to take action. I always stress with my clients (to the point they hear me in their head, even when I'm not there!)— "focus on the inputs and the outcome will take care of itself".

# 2 DIET

You might have tried diets before, seen results and lost some weight to begin with, but eventually end up heavier than when you began. This happens because most diets don't teach the fundamentals of what you need to do to lose weight and consistently keep it off.

If you've ever tracked points, counted your syns, or had shakes and meal replacements, they all have one thing in common: you're eating less calories than normal. That is the reason that all these seemingly different diets and plans lead to weight loss. There really is no magic formula. Success in weight loss is a simple mathematical equation. The only way to see successful weight loss is to get this formula right.

This is great news for you, because when you do, it becomes simple to understand and hit your weight loss goals; without deprivation, starving yourself, and getting bored on another 'diet'. When you understand how it works it is much simpler, and more flexible, than you might imagine.

"But I've tried everything, what if this doesn't work?" I understand— I too had tried almost every diet going. When I got the help that I needed, I started to implement it myself, and later with my many clients, I found that it actually works. In fact, it's very simple and even enjoyable. You might not believe me right now, but by the end of this chapter, if you commit to giving it a try for a few weeks, you will start to see changes.

## Losing Weight Doesn't Have To Be Complicated

There's an enemy out there fighting you on your weight loss journey. This enemy is the diet industry. The truth is, they don't want to see you succeed. They want you to fail because weight loss is a billion-dollar industry that makes more money from you the more diets you try, and the longer you stay on the cycle of endless dieting.

It's not your fault if you've been on a diet before and not lost weight. There are so many different diets and plans out there. It's confusing and an easy way for the diet industry to make money from your failure— by contradicting themselves, making it complicated, and secretive. The lack of simplicity in the industry is one of the biggest struggles people face. The reason that obesity and being overweight is such a problem in the UK and the USA is because people can't see which way is which. They're bamboozled by daily conflicting information and 'new research' saying to 'do this' today and 'do that' tomorrow.

When you walk back through the church hall doors for your fifth go at diet club the leader's eyes light up because they're thinking, "ooh, you're back, you're back". It's just more money for them. When you succeed and don't go any longer, they don't get paid.

I've done every single diet going, many of them multiple times, and many of them worked brilliantly at the time. You will lose weight if you follow the plan, but what they don't teach you, is how to continue keeping the weight off for the long term.

I have a friend who twice each year goes to one specific diet club because she gets to eat a lot of food when she follows this plan. Then a few months later she goes to the next one, where she can eat anything, as long as she watches how much she has. Meanwhile she keeps hopping between new diet plans every few months, often gaining more weight back than when she started. I'll ask the question, is that being successful? If you lose weight for a couple of weeks, then gain it back, did the diet work? Would you classify it as successful if you're still doing that at over seventy years of age, like my friend?

Would you not rather lose the weight and learn about how your body works? Find out what works for you, how you can change things when you're not seeing the results you want, and how you can create sustainable habits to maintain your weight, rather than yo-yoing up and down.

In this book we're going to simplify weight loss into a system that is easy to follow. Some of the straightforward advice you probably already know such as the Government guidelines which are things like: eat five portions of fruit and vegetables a day, drink more water, walk 10,000 steps. These recommendations are a great place to start. It doesn't have to be this big, complex thing where you're counting points, working out syn values, or living on powdered shakes. Simple is effective.

This **is not** for you if you…

- Are looking for a quick fix.
- Think you must live off rabbit food, dust, and air.
- Think you must spend hours in the gym, battling the treadmill.
- Want to go back to diet club because you've tried it before and it works well.
- Are looking for rapid weight loss because you have a party or event coming up in two weeks.
- Want to jump on the bandwagon of another diet merry-go-round.

This **is** for you if you…

- Have tried every diet going and are ready for the 'no-diet' formula.
- Want to enjoy real food, without giving up your favourite pizza or wine.
- Have a busy life, and want a simple solution.
- Can spare thirty minutes, three times per week.
- Are ready to commit to yourself with Project You.

## Why Make It Simple?

Having done so many diets over the years, I think I speak from authority on the experience of dieting. Every time you're looking at another new weight loss attempt you get that sense of, "oh God, I've got to try again, what if it doesn't work?".

When you figure out not only what to do, but more importantly *how* to do it (this is what I want to share in this book), it's much simpler than you may think. You will *know* that it works.

If I had a quid for every person that said, "I know what to do, I just don't seem to do it", I'd be rich! This book is not another diet quick fix. It's about how to find and implement a plan that works; not only this week but that is sustainable for life.

This plan which I call the 'no-diet formula' looks at making two or three small changes to your lifestyle every week, to build sustainable habits that are going to lead to weight loss, more energy, increased confidence and keeping those pounds off. The plan is designed to be effective in the short-term, but to really maximize success in the long-term by creating a new set of habits that make it 'easy' to maintain your results.

When you go along to a slimming club or you buy a plan on the internet, all those things point to different reasons for why you gained weight. They can't all be right. We will look at exactly what is and what is not important to worry about when you're trying to lose weight or live a healthier lifestyle.

When you try and do everything at once, as advocated by most plans out there, it's just not sustainable. By making two to three small changes every week, which you can commit to no matter how busy you are, and whatever your lifestyle looks like, you can see sustainable change.

If you've got to cook fancy food, change everything you do in your daily routine, restock everything in your cupboard, get to the gym four or five times a week; it's just not feasible. It's too much. Forget about all that. If you can commit to making a few small changes each you, you can commit to losing weight.

As you're reading this, you might be thinking that making small changes every week doesn't sound like enough to see big results…

It's not going to happen in one week, but over a period of time many small changes adds up to a lot of total change. My client, Maddy had a conversation with somebody who said, "wow, you've lost a lot of weight, you look amazing". Her reply, "oh, it's been really easy, I've just made a couple of small changes". That's how she thought until she started talking about it. Then she realized that over a period of twelve weeks, two or three changes each week adds up to a huge amount of change.

She told me, "I couldn't believe how much had changed, but it hasn't felt like I've done anything difficult or I have really done that much, because a couple of changes every week is really easy. In twelve weeks, I've done what I've been trying to do for the last five years".

## Making Your First Small Changes

Let's look at what these changes might look like.

One change will be something to do with your food and nutrition. One will be around exercise and one will be around lifestyle.

Remember, making these little changes isn't about getting results quickly. It's about making lasting change. If you've ever been on a diet before and seen results quickly, you've usually restricted or starved yourself, and inevitably you put all the weight back on as soon as you stop doing that.

You don't want to get back on that cycle of losing and regaining the weight forever— let's get you off that train!

## Action Steps

1. Take photos of your food so you're aware of what you're eating— it will really open your eyes to what you're doing, and it is so easy to track.

    This isn't about being judgmental but simply observational. My clients often tell me how surprised they are by some of their food choices, both positively and negatively.

2. Drink more water. If you don't drink any, drink one litre. If you drink one litre, then drink one-and-a-half litres, etc. It's the single easiest, quickest win for weight loss.

When you stay properly hydrated, you'll have more energy and less hunger cravings too.

## The Simple Mathematical Equation For Weight Loss

I want to share with you the key equation for weight loss. I'm afraid it's not some big secret that I had to trek through the Amazon rainforest to learn from a guru who required a blood sacrifice to reveal this ancient wisdom.. It's a very simple math's formula that you probably learnt at school.
If you're gaining weight— you're eating too many calories (for your age, shape, height, gender, and activity level).

If your weight is stable— you're eating the right number of calories (for your age, shape, height, gender, and activity level).

To lose weight you need to eat fewer calories than you currently are, if right now you are maintaining or gaining weight.

Calories count. Even though some people will tell you they don't. It is a scientific fact that they do. Having said that, by making small changes, increasing your activity levels, and putting a little bit of thought into what you do daily, you can start to lose weight, and keep it off, without needing to be obsessed about calories.

Ultimately, you will need to know how many calories you are eating, but it is not by any stretch the first thing you need to do. You can manipulate your calorie intake without being obsessive about it or counting every little thing, every single day.

While you might lose weight on this or that diet, the underlying mechanism of ALL successful weight loss is a calorie deficit. The different diets are just different ways of achieving it.

The other day I googled 'free online diet plans' and there were 170 *million* results. Today, I overheard people talking about how we're getting more obese as a nation, childhood obesity is rising, etc. While the information is there, and anybody can find and follow these diets, what they do not account for is that while we all lose weight in the same way, we have different lifestyles, different needs, and different understanding.

A lot of people say, "I know what I need to do, I just need to do it". Sometimes people have all the information, they know how to successfully lose weight and could tell someone else how to do it, but they don't do it themselves. Why is that?

We need to break it down, not for greater understanding, but so we can implement and move forward. More information is not always helpful. It only works if you do it. Sometimes simplicity is the answer.

All those 170 million diet plans say something different. The information web is keeping you stuck 'learning'. Instead, ask what you can do today to get started?

Implementing a plan brings results. Doing some of the right things is better than doing nothing at all, even if what you're doing is not perfect.

Remember, the simple equation for weight loss is calories in versus calories out. You need to be in a calorie deficit for your age, height, gender, and activity level; to lose weight. That is really all there is to it. Everything else is simply a different way of achieving that goal.

## A Simple Way To Reduce Calories...

The diet industry confuses things for you on purpose, because they don't want you to know how to lose weight on your own. A diet puts you in a calorie deficit, which you need to be in to lose weight. That's about it. I don't want to get too scientific with you, because we're trying to avoid overwhelm, but this is essentially what you need to do. Consume less energy than you expend.

There are some things that you need to be aware of, to make this happen. A lot of people know what they're doing. One of the things that they say for example is, "I know my portion sizes are too big". In that case, a simple way to reduce calories is to reduce your portion sizes. That's a really easy way to start your diet plan— by simply looking at controlling your caloric intake with reduced portion sizes.

Portion sizes have increased over the years. If you look at the size of an average dinner plate, your Granny's dinner plate compared to the size of your dinner plate now; your dinner plate will be significantly larger.

Nowadays when people go out for a meal they often judge whether the meal was good by the amount of food they got, not by the quality of food. "Oh, it was really good because it had lots of food and big portion sizes", is the first thing people say, instead of "it was delicious, and it tasted good".

How much food you get has become a marker for the quality and value a restaurant provides. We need to take a step back and consider whether looking at things from this perspective is helping or hurting us.

## What Kind of Portions Should We Be Aiming For?

The government guidelines have a portion size guide which you can measure with your hands. That's a quick and simple test you can use to see whether the portion sizes you're eating are too big or even too small.

Specifically, they say that you should consume a piece of protein the size of the palm of your hand, which is one portion. You should have one portion of protein at each meal. Focusing on getting enough protein into your diet is a good place to start. We'll look at all the macronutrients later in the book and why they're important. Protein is the most important when it comes to weight loss and the first place to focus.

The point I'm making here is that this can be very simple. Don't be like a lot of people saying "I know I eat too much. My portion sizes are too big". You have very straightforward guidelines for measuring and controlling your portions. All you have to do is follow them.

This is a quick way that you can look at how much you're eating. Although it's not the most scientific way, it is a good starting point to get a feeling of control over your diet. The good thing about portion sizes based on your palm is that everybody's hand is a different size. It's a rough indication for you specifically based on your body size and shape.

You can also take pictures. Be honest with yourself by documenting exactly what you're eating in photographic form. As the saying goes, "what gets measured gets managed". Simply taking a photograph of your meals— without trying to change anything— brings so much awareness to your diet, it naturally shines a light on what you might need to change. After looking at your photos, simply ask yourself and be honest— how much are you eating?

Aim for one palm of protein at each meal and loads of vegetables, or a bit of fruit on the side. We'll get deeper in to what to eat later in the book, but that is my simple recommendation that you can action now. Increasing your awareness of what you are doing will often bring results, without even needing a strict plan to follow.

Go to www.lisaalicoach.com/portions to see appropriate portion sizes.

## Not All Calories Are Created Equal

I've talked about how important creating a calorie deficit is. That it's a simple mathematical equation to lose weight, by expending more calories than you consume. Having said that, does this mean you can eat ten donuts which might be say 1,500 calories? Would that be good for you and give you all the nutrients that you need? No.

Not all calories are created equal. You get more bang for your buck if you look at the source of what you're eating too. What I mean by the source is that you could have a pretty good meal for about 250-300 calories— a piece of chicken, a small portion of rice, and plenty of vegetables. That same number of calories might be a single Mars bar. Not all calories are created equal and eating the more nutrient dense food is going to give you much better health, more energy, and be more filling.

When you base all your meals around a good source of protein, and what I call 'single ingredient foods' (meat, fish, eggs, vegetables, fruit, rice, etc.) not only will you get results quicker, but you will be giving your body all the nutrients that it needs to feel great, be energized, and improve your health.

That's not to say you can't enjoy meals out. Of the twenty-one meals in a week, there's lots of opportunity to make those great choices that fuel your body, and still have room for a few things that you want to enjoy. You don't have to be 'strict' 100% of the time, but you should focus on eating healthful, nutritious foods most of the time.

## What Gets Measured Gets Managed

You might not actually be aware of how much you're eating or how big your portion sizes are. By simply snapping a picture of what you eat, you start to get an idea. Take pictures and then compare them against standard portion sizes. You'll get a bit more of an indication about whether you are overeating or not. This is a starting point aimed at increasing awareness.

Step one is to start identifying how much you're eating, which we've looked at above. Step two is to start tracking in My Fitness Pal to get a more accurate indication of precisely how much you're eating. My Fitness Pal is a free app that you can download onto your smart phone or computer, to help you track how many calories you're eating every day. You can download from Google Play or the App Store and it will give you simple instructions on how to set it up. It's the most useful little app for weight loss. It makes keeping track of what you're doing a breeze.

Of course, it is not always 100% accurate, but it is a meaningful way to gather some data. It's very self-explanatory. Just track your food for a couple of days. You can log your food by searching in the search engine or if you've got something in a packet, you can scan the barcode on the packaging. Do that before you eat, not afterwards, when you risk forgetting to do it. Start tracking your calories for just two days. Do one day during the week, and one at the weekend.

You can scan the barcode and check most chain restaurants for meals in the search function inside the app. When you're at the office canteen or somewhere else where you did not prepare the food and don't necessarily know the ingredients— have a look through the search function. A piece of chicken breast might range from 120 calories to 250 calories depending on size. I suggest going for the midway point of what is in the app. If you don't know the size and weight of something, overestimate it rather than underestimate it. It will work both ways and ultimately balance out.

## Using Your Food Data

The first point here is that you don't want to be overwhelmed. To begin with, get used to tracking your calories with My Fitness Pal. Get an indication of how much you're eating, and what types of food you're eating. It's about increasing awareness and being honest. The more data you have at hand, the more accurate a picture you have of what is going on.

Not that people are dishonest, but they probably don't know exactly what they're doing. They've never considered how much they eat and tracked it this way. It's very easy for things to slip in— a biscuit in the office, a Frappuccino in the morning— that you forget you had— leaving you with the impression you've been eating healthy and should lose weight, but extra calories have slipped in which you're not accounting for. This leaves you not losing weight, and frustrated because you don't understand why.

Back to the simple equation; its calories in versus calories out. If you don't know how much you're eating, you don't know whether you're overeating or you're in a calorie deficit. The first step is understanding how many calories you're eating. Any changes you make can only follow from an accurate picture of where you are right now.

You might have tried a low-calorie diet before, and feel like it didn't work for you? What all these diet clubs and programmes will not look at, is your personal lifestyle. It's not about eating low calories, but rather eating the right amount for you.

If you eat too low calorie, it won't work long term. I've had clients where the first thing we had to do was get them to eat more, because they're not eating enough calories; they're eating only 1,000 calories a day. I would never, ever, suggest anybody eats less than 1,200 calories a day. Even that is still low for most people. Eating too low calorie is simply not sustainable. It makes you hungry, miserable, and you won't continue doing it for long.

If you lower your calories to the right amount and find yourself hungry a lot, then look at the quality of food you're eating. Look for foods that are going to keep you fuller for longer. The food that's going to fill you up the most is protein like lean meat, fish, eggs, cottage cheese, Greek yoghurt, milk, tuna, salmon, prawns. These proteins will keep you feeling full for longer when you make them the base of each meal.

Women often don't eat enough protein. It's the last thing they go to when they're creating a meal. We need to make the switch to seeing protein as the most important part of your meals.

Don't worry that too much protein is bad for you. You're more likely to get kidney failure from drinking too much alcohol and eating chocolate biscuits. (Which, by the way, you can still eat chocolate biscuits if you want. It's just going to take a little longer to reach your goal if you're eating chocolate biscuits on a regular basis. Nothing is off limits, but everything needs to be honestly accounted for.)

Government guidelines suggest the average woman needs 2,000 calories for weight maintenance, a man needs 2,500 calories. 1lb of fat is about 3,500 calories of energy. If you eat 500 calories less per day for seven days this equals 3,500-calorie deficit per week— which would mean you set your calories at 1,500 per day as a woman, or 2,000 as a man— and you will be in a calorie deficit to lose 1lb of fat per week. This is just a simple rule of thumb, there is a much more technical way, but for now we are focused on making this simple and easy to implement.

If you're using My Fitness Pal be aware that it does have limitations. If you say you want to lose two pounds per week. It might set your calories as low as 1,200 calories or less. That is too low for most people. My clients typically start on 1,700 calories per day and that is quite a lot of food, especially when you focus on protein and vegetables at every meal, which have more nutrients and less calories. Eating that kind of healthy, nutritious food is a simple way of reducing calories without thinking about it too much and while still having enough food volume to feel satisfied.

## Being Restrictive Leads to Failure

Most of us have been on a diet before, and typically we try to change everything at once. We think that when we go on a diet we can only eat salad, or we can't have this, and we can't do that. We can't go out, mustn't eat that. It's all a very negative connotation toward dieting, based on restriction.

It's setting ourselves up to fail. People say things like, "well, I've got to be in the right head space before I start a diet", thinking that they're not going to be able to eat what they want whilst they're on a diet. They must prepare themselves mentally for the restrictive torture that is coming. Does that sound like a good experience for you?

That's why very quickly, after just a couple of weeks, you start craving things that you're not eating. You start craving whatever it is you like, whether it's chocolate, cake, take away pizza with the husband, a glass of wine.

You can use willpower to resist these cravings for a while, but you get to a certain point and something will happen along the way that throws you off track. You 'cave in' and eat the 'bad foods'.

It might be that you go for a night out with the girls, you drink too much, and you think, "oh, I've blown it now". You wobble, fall off the horse and start to think you're a failure. It might be that your weight plateaus because you've been too restrictive and you're not eating enough calories, then you think, "well, this doesn't work. I've been really, really good and I've not lost any weight". So, you quit and quickly balloon back up.

Truth is, it's not about being good and bad. Food is just food. It's simply a case of managing the choices we make and focusing on doing things that serve us moving towards our goals. People say "I've been really good all week. I've only eaten salad, I've not eaten any bread, not had any chocolate, I didn't go out at the weekend. I've been really good".

I don't believe this way of thinking helps. 'Really good' is helping the old lady next door do her shopping— not avoiding bread. That is just a choice of what you are eating. Or people say the opposite, "I've been bad, I was good all week, but on the weekend, I went out and had a takeaway, then there was some chocolate left in the cupboard. I'd forgotten it was there, but I found it, so I ate it and then I've had a couple of glasses of wine to wash it down. I've been really bad". Again, eating a piece of chocolate does not make you 'bad'. Being bad is killing somebody, not eating a piece of chocolate.

It's about understanding and accepting that food is just food. It's a choice you make, it's not about good or bad. The sooner you start thinking, "I'm going to make a choice that serves me and takes me towards my goals", the easier it becomes.

This may sound easy for me to say, but truly letting go of the thought of being good and bad around food makes such a huge difference for my clients. As Paula said "I've now learned that I have the power to make good dietary decisions without existing just on rabbit food— and I can even have treats— and get the results I want.

The right 'diet' is based on having everything in moderation. It's not about doing everything spot on all through the week and then thinking that you've blown it because you had a piece of cake at the weekend. It's just doing things moderately when you're trying to lose weight. Enjoying a small piece of cake, not eating half of the cake (and not even enjoying it because you're just binging).

It might be that you choose to eat two meals early in the day which are lower in calories, and then you enjoy an evening meal with your family. It might be that you say, "I know that I'm going out on Saturday, so I'm going to make sure I leave some extra calories spare in my weekly calories. That way I'm still in the deficit for the week overall and will still see results".

Even if you were doing that and happened to overeat on your night out or at the weekend, it's not the end of the world. Just get back on track. That's where people go wrong. They think it's the end of the world if they go off track. One night won't be the defining moment of what happens over one week or one month. It's not what you do once a week that matters. It's what you do consistently and regularly throughout the week that counts

This idea of weekly or monthly calories instead of getting too caught up in each day can by illustrated by the fact that most of my clients lose weight over Christmas, New Years, and Thanksgiving. One of them last year had the same breakfast every day. It struck me that she had this great option for breakfast that worked for her. Then she mixed other things up and enjoyed herself, had a drink and some good food later in the day. She didn't need to deprive herself, she just managed her intake and controlled the things she ate earlier in the day. In the end, you're still in a deficit overall.

You simply work around whatever situation you find yourself facing. Plan how many times you want to go out, how important it is to enjoy yourself and then account for it. Some parties are more important than others. You don't have to splurge every time, but when you want to go out, simply account for it by lowering calories the rest of the day or week, to balance out and end up at your goal number of calories for the day or week.

## You Will Crave What You Restrict

When you give something up, you start to crave it. When you think you can't have something, you crave it even more so. "I can't have that, so I want it". As soon as you deny yourself something, as soon as you say, "I can't have this, I'm on a diet", it's like saying to your kids, "stop switching the light on and off. Don't do that". They'll inevitably do it even more. As soon as you try to condition yourself with that negativity of "can't", "mustn't", "shouldn't", you'll want it even more.

If you want something, have it, but make sure you really enjoy it, if you know it's perhaps not the best choice for taking you towards your goals.

When you're thinking, "I've been really spot on with my diet, it's Thursday afternoon and I've got a low energy slump. Somebody just bought some cake and I really would like some cake", first, work out if you do really want that cake. Just sit quietly for a minute and ask, do you want that cake? What's more important, eating the cake or continuing with some of the good habits you're starting to implement and the weight you're losing?

If you do really want it, that's fine. Eat it mindfully and consciously, enjoy and savour every mouthful. If you have something, and feel like you want to keep eating more, first wait for twenty minutes and decide if you really do want more. Have a glass of water. If you still want it, go ahead, but eat every mouthful consciously, deliberately, and make sure you enjoy it.

It's not about self-control. It's about repeating the same process of self-awareness. If you really enjoyed it and you want to have more, that's ok. Simply ask, do you really want another bit? Or are you satisfied? Did you enjoy it? Are you full and satisfied already?

The enemy is not eating 'bad foods'. It is eating mindlessly. I did a lot of mindless eating with the chocolate biscuits at the weekend. Two would've been plenty. It's that mindless eating that creeps up on you. Sometimes people say, "I can sit and eat a whole packet of biscuits and I get to the end of it, I don't know how I've managed to eat the whole packet, but by the end of it I feel sick".

If instead you took yourself and sat down, maybe put the biscuits on the plate in front of you, ate them slowly and consciously; you'd be full quite quickly. You wouldn't want more than a couple, certainly not the whole packet, and you would probably enjoy it a lot more by eating consciously. Not to mention, being able to stop, to control yourself; you'd probably have a lot more respect for yourself.

There's a lot of people that struggle with emotional eating. The key is giving yourself permission to do it. Acceptance is what it's about. If you want to do it, give yourself permission to do it. Don't say, "I want! I want!", just sit down and say, "OK, I'm going to give myself permission to do this".

When you have permission to do it, that might stop you wanting to do it. Even if not, you will remain emotionally neutral, rather than beating yourself up.

The next time you find yourself craving a certain food that isn't the best choice, follow this simple sequence:

1. Sit for a minute and think if you *really* want the food.

2. If yes, give yourself permission to eat it - you control what you are doing, not the food.

3. Savour every single mouthful. Eat it slowly and consciously and enjoy it, without guilt or shame.

## If You're Overly Restrictive...

If you're overly restrictive and eat too little, you're starving your body. If your body thinks it's going to starve, you won't lose the fat you're hoping to. When you do these crash diets and very low-calorie diets; yes, you might lose weight very quickly to begin, but your weight will soon plateau because you're not eating enough. Your body will hold onto its energy stores (body fat) as a protection against starvation.

Then you become frustrated because you don't understand why you're not losing weight when you're trying so hard, and you're hungry all the time. Not to mention, you're just not treating your body or yourself very kindly.

Undereating will slow your metabolism down, making it harder to lose weight in the future. In fact, it makes it harder to just maintain where you are. You end up having to eat less, just to stay where you are; after your metabolism has slowed down due to aggressive dieting. The more you eat the right amount of food; your body will recover and learn to burn off the excess fat without having to starve.

I did a shakes and chocolate bar diet once. You have a shake for breakfast, chocolate bar for lunch, and soup for dinner. They all come together in a pack. I did it for about 4 days. While doing it I was talking to my mum and said to her that I was bloody ravenous. I was supposed to go for another couple of days just having this shake, soup, and bar of chocolate. My mother said, "You're hungry darling, do you think you should eat some food?".

I didn't want to break the diet, but she was right. I got off the phone and luckily had some chicken in the fridge. I made some chicken and vegetables and it was such a relief. I couldn't do it any longer and binged the rest of that day. The beast was released, and I ate everything. I couldn't go back to the horrible packet of soup again.

Have you ever been through this cycle? I, for one, never plan to do that again! Thankfully, you don't need to.

## You Can Eat Whatever You Want, But...

I don't want to give the wrong impression here. Some people think, when they hear that you can eat whatever you want, "oh that's great, I don't have to change anything". For better health, you need to achieve better balance. Simple foods with few ingredients, generally what you might consider 'healthy foods' should be the bulk of your diet. Getting that balance and moderation where, if you're eating right most of the time, a 'treat' will not cause you any harm allows you flexibility and freedom to enjoy what you are doing. You don't have to restrict yourself because that will be unsustainable. Nobody will restrict themselves forever.

Quality of food is important. You may have heard the maxim; *"eat shit, feel shit"*. For feeling good, having lots of energy, and being as healthy as possible, you want to eat healthy food. It's not just about what helps you to lose weight, but also what fuels you to feel good throughout your day.

But what *is* healthy food? Single ingredient food is going to be much healthier. If it's in a packet and you can't read all the ingredients, its likely not very healthy. That doesn't mean you can't ever have a donut. It's simply a choice of eating single ingredient foods more often.

Base your diet around things like chicken, fish, apples, bananas, green beans, broccoli, rice, potatoes or plant based protein. Things that are highly processed are not going to be as healthy. That doesn't mean you can't eat them, but they probably shouldn't be the foundation of your diet.

There is science that says if you're in a calorie deficit, you will lose weight. That's true, but it's only looking at one aspect (weight loss). We should also think about fueling your body, being healthy, and feeling great as well.

Say you want to eat a donut for breakfast; and that donut you have for breakfast is 250 calories. Firstly, it's full of sugar. It's going to send your blood sugar rocketing. It will give you an immediate high, but you're going to crash about 10:00 in the morning, being left lethargic and hungry.

Secondly, for 250 calories, you can eat a lot more food that's going to fill you up, and make you feel good. It's going to be better for your body and give you more energy— keeping you fuller for longer, so you may not need the 10am snacks.

What we eat is not just about losing weight. There is also the consideration of what some foods are doing inside your body. If you always eat heavily processed foods you're not giving yourself the best nutrients and energy. Donuts are OK occasionally— I'm not saying eliminate them completely, but if you make that the basis of your diet, you will get hungry regularly. Maybe you can still lose weight if you manage to not eat too many, but you won't feel great.

Looking only at weight loss is short-term thinking— it's about giving your health a better shot too. Healthy foods are single ingredient foods, but it doesn't mean it has to be bland or that all your food must be single ingredient foods prepared at home. It's about having good quality foods that serve your health most of the time.

Make the base of your diet the right things, and you can enjoy yourself a little around the edges. I'm repeating this to really get the message home. Dieting is not an 'all or nothing' equation, but you should be focused on having healthful foods that fuel you and gives you lots of nutrients.

Concentrate on eating good sources of protein, lots of fresh fruit and vegetables, good sources of carbohydrates and quality sources of fats (more information on what these are in the next section). Add in lots of herbs and spices to make it tasty and exciting. A lot of people think they don't have time to cook healthy food, or to prepare their own food. I understand that— I used to live Monday to Friday in a hotel room while I was working on projects, but here's the thing - I think that's a fallacy.

If you've got a microwave, it's not that difficult. You can buy microwave rice, it takes two minutes to cook, and that's a good source of carbohydrates. You can buy pre-cooked chicken, chop that up and stick it in your rice. You can buy pre-packed, vegetables for the microwave. It's not difficult. If you're at home, it's just as easy sticking the oven on and waiting for twenty minutes for a pizza to cook, as it is to put chicken in there, a baked potato, and wait for the same twenty minutes.

I make things like curries, chili con carne, things with sauces on, stir fry's. It doesn't have to be bland, but it doesn't have to be complicated either. You don't need to eat a quinoa and pomegranate salad (unless you like it). You can just make a nice salad and put a tasty dressing on it, or simply top it with olive oil. Even if you use a shop bought dressing, it doesn't really matter. If most of your food is coming from better sources you will lose weight and see an increase in health, energy, etc.

As my client Meg said, "I never took care of myself. It was too easy an excuse to go out the door and not make breakfast, but actually it's just as easy to scramble some eggs in the microwave as it is to pick something up from the coffee shop".

It's a choice. It's not just weight loss but the choice is; do you just want to do this to lose weight, or do you want to increase your energy, have more focus, feel great inside and out, and know that you're treating your body kindly? Do you want to give yourself the best chance to live longer?

Another thing people often ask about is alcohol. Something that a lot of people turn to, along with comfort eating, as a source of release, to de-stress. I think it's about making those choices and asking if you can make some better swaps or just assessing what you're doing. Alcohol is very high in calories. If you are going out at the weekend and drinking a couple of bottles of wine, that might be impacting your ability to stay in a calorie deficit for the entire week.

If you want to have alcohol, that's fine. It's not about saying that you shouldn't have alcohol. If you want to have it you can, but perhaps you could make better choices around what you drink, how much, and how often. Start looking at *why* you're drinking and in what situations you turn to alcohol.

One of my clients used to struggle with alcohol when her step son came to visit. The relationship was so stressful. He came in to the family and disrupted everything; she would just turn to wine for the whole weekend he was there. I felt sorry for her. I felt sorry for the step-son too, because he clearly has some problems going on.

Ultimately, she sat down with her husband-to-be and they thrashed it out, getting the truth on the table. She didn't do it in a judgmental way, but it made such a huge difference. She realized that she was just drinking to cope, and that there's other ways you can cope with stress. She also realized that it was impacting her efforts to lose weight and leaving her frustrated, long after the step-son had left.

Like everything else, alcohol is simply another choice we make. One thing that people don't understand about alcohol, or they don't want to admit, is that it is toxic. Your body will get rid of the alcohol first, before it starts burning fat, because alcohol is poisonous in the blood stream.

Aside from the calorie load in alcohol, we also need to be aware that perhaps if we've had a few too many, we might not make the best choices in other things. We might hit the box of chocolates, the burger or whatever; because our inhibitions are lowered.

That's not to say you should never drink. However, if you say that you only drink three or four times a week, that's half of the week and will impact on your ability to lose weight. It's coming down to choices again. It's not saying to never do it, that you're never going to go out and have too much to drink, but it's looking at how you want to meet your goals and asking if this going to be the best choice for you?

If you want to lose weight, you need to be in a calorie deficit, and alcohol is generally not going to help you achieve that.

## It's Not What You Do Once...

It's not what you do once a week, it's what you do consistently the rest of the time that will determine your outcomes. People think they've blown everything because they go out once, or have one high-calorie meal, one bar of chocolate; and then they go off the rails. They give up because they 'ruined their diet'. That's not how it works. It's what you do with consistency and commitment over a longer period of time that makes the changes you're looking for and becomes habit forming.

Sometimes life will happen, maybe you have a wedding, a big event, or you're going on holiday. You want to enjoy the event, but you also want to keep losing weight and not get thrown off track with your goals.

I've got three strategies for such occasions. It's up to you which you pick. Having these strategies in place addresses the fact that holidays are always going to happen. Christmas is always going to happen. Your birthday is always going to come along. There's always going to be a party or an event. It's a case of picking the strategy that works for you.

Do you want to carry on losing weight? Do you want to maintain your weight? Or do you want to say screw it - I call it the 'fuck it' strategy - and say I'm going to eat and drink what I want and I'm dealing with the consequences afterwards?

If you pick strategy one, to continue losing weight, you carry on doing what you're doing and maybe increase your exercise, while you have a bit more of the food that you fancy. Maybe you stick with your healthy breakfast, healthy lunch, and then in the evening you have what you'd like. Whether you want to have a dessert or whatever, you let go of inhibition and enjoy yourself. Simply add in a bit more exercise as well, to burn a few extra calories. Keep things on track the rest of the week and balance out your weekly calories to continue losing weight.

Strategy two: if you want to maintain, you'd just enjoy yourself a little more, while keeping 80% of your routine, and still doing your exercise. Switch off from being 'strict' but keep your eating conscious— don't binge on food you don't really want. Make a conscious choice to eat a bit, enjoy it, and then stop when you've had enough.

Strategy three, you just enjoy yourself and worry about it when you come home. Enjoy yourself while you're in the moment and prepare for it, knowing you might gain some weight. Be ok that you will probably gain a couple of pounds, because you're committed to getting back to normal and losing them again the following week.

Which strategy is right for you? That's your choice. Ultimately this all comes down to choice. It's not about being good or bad, not about going on a diet, not about failing or succeeding. It's about making choices.

Nobody can tell you what you want to do— whether you want to maintain your weight, lose weight or you don't want to bother worrying about it while you enjoy yourself. Then you must deal with the outcome.

I used to not believe you could lose weight over Christmas and New Year. I didn't think it was possible because of everything going on. I had this conversation with my coach when I was first going through my own transformation, and I ended up losing two pounds that Christmas. I really didn't think it was possible, because I had never done it before, but after that conversation I realised it was simply the choices I made. There's no right answer for what you *should* do, it is just what you choose to do. We all have choices in life, we choose them every day.

This happened to me last week: My alarm didn't go off, because my phone was updating, which reset the phone. My husband's alarm went off and woke us up later than I normally get up. I've been getting up earlier, so I can get to the gym and get started with my day early. It really threw me off my schedule getting up later.

Now, if you were going to work in an office and your alarm didn't go off, would you go, "well, I'm not going to bother to go today". Probably not. You make that choice that you still get up and go to work. Why would it be different choosing to get up and go to the gym? What would you do?

When it comes to choosing to go to the gym or not, it's not that one is right, and one is wrong. Simply make the choice and stick to it. Own it.

If you choose to restrict food, you can miss out on vital nutrients. People think if they just cut out carbs, which is a very popular one for women, they will lose weight. When you cut entire food groups out of your diet you're missing out on vital nutrients that your body needs. Not to mention, they taste good. You want to eat food that tastes good because when you're only eating very bland, repetitive food, restricting yourself; you will quickly get bored and come to dislike your diet.

A couple of people told me something like, "I have quite a good diet. I cook things from scratch. I like cooking, I've got all the diet books going". When you drill down into it, start recording your intake, being aware— but not being obsessed—about what you do or don't do, it's amazing how quickly you can see things. Perhaps— and this is not a judgement— you're not as accurate as you might think. When you're aware of it, and you take photos of your food, you realise that the perception of what you're eating might be off.

They think that they eat well. Once they consciously look at what they're doing and look at the choices they make, quite quickly they realize that perhaps that's not the case. My client Maddy said it to me when we began working together, "I eat quite well really". When she started taking pictures of what she ate for the first few days of her food diary, she went on to say, "actually, I don't eat as well as I thought I did. I tend to go into Starbucks and grab a sandwich for breakfast with cheese in it, along with a large latte. Then at lunch time I go out again and have lots of carbs. I do this, and I do that…".

It's a case of being aware of what you're doing. While you might make a healthy meal in the evening (and that might not be every day because you might go out a few days) what is happening the rest of the time? You might have twenty-one meals a week, but if you're going out three nights, then you only make a healthy dinner four nights a week. Then you have a cereal bar for breakfast and grab a sandwich off the shelf in Tesco's for lunch every day. You're only eating four out of the twenty-one meals you think are healthy.

Remember you want to look at it as if you've got twenty-one meals, you want to be going the other way around to lose weight. Eating healthy, preparing your own food for seventeen of those, and then maybe picking something up, or eating out for the other four.

Using this model, you are making healthy choices most of the time. Then you have flexibility around the small percentage of meals to do what you please or take it easy when eating out and you want to enjoy yourself.

## Nutrition Recap

Be aware of what you're eating. Take pictures of your meals for two- three days. Don't try and change what you're doing because if you try and change it before you know what you have been doing, you won't have any idea of what is going on. To begin, just take some time to look at it. Look at the portion sizes. Do your portion sizes seem big, small, or moderate? How many meals do you grab on the go? How many meals do you cook from scratch? How many times do you go out to eat?

Get awareness of where you are right now. If you don't know where you are right now, you can't know what you need to do to get where you want to be. Get the awareness of what you're doing right now, by tracking and taking photos.

Once you've got that awareness, then you can download My Fitness Pal. Start by putting in your goal— for the average woman— 1,700 calories a day. This is a 300-calorie deficit, now begin tracking your food.

Finally, here is the first simple change to make. People totally underestimate how much water they need. One of the single simplest, cheapest, easiest, quickest, most effective weight loss methods is to drink more water.

People say, "Oh yeah, I know I should drink more water, but I don't". Change that. The impact of being properly hydrated cannot be underestimated. Track your water intake on My Fitness Pal and increase how much water you're drinking. If you don't drink any water, start by drinking one litre a day, get used to drinking one litre a day, and then build up from there.

Next look at eating protein as the base of every meal. If you have protein at every meal, and are meeting your calorie goal, you will lose weight.

Just those two simple things will make everything else happen that you need to do to lose weight, have more energy, and feel great.

## Action Steps

1. Take photos of your food for 3 days and assess what you're eating, along with portion sizes.

2. Drink more water every day and record how much you are drinking.

3. Eat protein (meat, fish, eggs, cheese, beans, pulses, lentils, tofu etc.) at every meal.

4. Download My Fitness Pal and get tracking for an accurate picture.

# 3 EXERCISE

Exercise comes in many shapes, forms and fashions. It's not just spending hours in the gym pumping iron or plodding away on the treadmill. While we should be aware that exercise is a key component in a healthy lifestyle, it's a much smaller component than what you eat. Especially when it comes to weight loss. You may have heard that to lose weight, 80% will come down to what you eat, and 20% will be exercise.

As one of my clients said to me, think of exercise as bonus. The key is making sure that you get a good balance of both. Food that fills you up and fuels you well; along with exercise that you enjoy, can sustain, and gives you an endorphin rush to make you feel good.

Exercise is important for…

- Making you feel good.
- Improving your internal systems like heart and lungs - you can't see it, but you know it's important.
- Increasing your energy levels.
- Ultimately it will help change your body shape, become more toned, build more strength, or have the look that you desire.

Exercise is not about…

- Being the biggest component of your weight loss journey.
- Spending hours on the treadmill trying to burn extra calories.
- Wasting hours and hours in the gym every day.
- Being boring and monotonous.

- Replacing a healthy diet, or justification to eat high-calorie, unhealthy food.

The first thing I want to talk about is simple, low-level activity that burns calories. The technical term is non-exercise activity thermogenesis (NEAT). We've become very sedentary as a nation. When we were kids, we didn't have a remote control for the television. You had to get up and walk over to change the channel. My mum didn't have a car until I was eleven, so we walked everywhere. We would walk miles or occasionally we'd get on the bus, laden down with shopping and things. Play involved being outside running around, rather than sitting inside in front of a screen.

We have become a very sedentary society. We just don't move as much as we used to and people underestimate the importance of this change. If I may give you some simple advice; just move a bit more. Don't underestimate that every little bit of exercise makes an impact. I do things such as take the stairs rather than the lift. I go to the toilet upstairs instead of the one closer. They have stand up desks now, which I have just got, instead of sitting on my bum all day. Even things like doing the house work, fidgeting around, doing a bit of gardening, walking a little bit more. All those things add up and count for a lot.

If you don't move much you're just not burning as many calories. I'll use my husband as an example. When we were in London, he was always out working on site visits even though he officially worked in an office. He'd be on the building site, he'd go into London and be walking around all day. He was very rarely at his desk in the office. He was just out and about moving around and being active.

I think the single biggest change when we moved back to Hastings was that he became very sedentary. He'd go from upstairs to downstairs and sit at his desk all day working from home. That inevitably lead to weight gain.

To add more non-exercise activity into your life simply take the stairs, park the car a little bit further away, stand up and move around more. Don't send an email when you can get up and go to talk to someone. Go to the toilet on a different floor, walk to the copy machine a bit further away. You can pull the weeds out the garden, or whatever you like doing. There is no right or wrong here. It is simply unstructured physical activity that you enjoy or do without even noticing you're doing 'exercise'.

It won't give you the body of a Victoria's Secret supermodel, but it does count. It's not the only thing that will make a difference, but it will start to make a difference not only in your weight, but even more in how you feel and your energy levels.

Your body burns calories three different ways. One, you will burn calories regardless, just sitting, doing nothing. You need a certain number of calories to live. That's called your basal metabolic rate (BMR). The second way is simply eating food; you burn calories to digest food. This is known as the thermic effect of food (TEE). The third is specifically through exercise and activity. You should be aware that this is only a relatively small percentage (about 10% of the total), so we count exercise as a bonus, while focusing mostly on food intake to drive weight loss.

When my clients want to start doing more exercise, and they're not sure where to start, I simply ask them what they like to do? I always like to ask what they like doing, because there is no point in saying you've got to go to the gym five times a week if you don't like going to the gym. They're not going to be able to do that.

One of my clients went back to the gym for the first time while working with me and when she checked in at the desk they asked her, "do you know the last time you were here?". It was over 1,000 days previously. She made the choice to go back to the gym herself, I would never have pushed her to do that, as she clearly didn't enjoy it in the past if she hadn't been for nearly three years.

I'll simply ask my clients, what do you like doing? They might say, "I like swimming". Cool, when was the last time you went swimming? "Gosh, I can't remember". If you like swimming; go swimming.

If you used to really like your Zumba class, go and book a Zumba class. Do what you like doing. That's the most important thing. If you struggle for time, simply ask yourself, "can I commit to thirty minutes, or even just twenty minutes, three times a week?". Most people can, and you can just go for a walk if you don't want to do anything more than that. Get a pair of trainers on and walk. Maybe just ten minutes at lunchtime, ten minutes in the evening. Start to do something and build from there.

If you do no exercise at all right now, start with walking briskly for ten minutes every day. That is progress from doing nothing, and every little bit of progress helps. Decide what you like and make a commitment to go one more time than you did the previous week. Start building the habit of being active and worry about the 'best' exercise later.

## Exercise Recommendations

As an ideal start, I recommend three, thirty-minute sessions of exercise per week. Many people think that to be effective and lose weight, you've got to spend hours on the treadmill doing loads of cardio or lifting weights. Ultimately both have benefits and you should have a combination of strength training and cardio in your exercise routine, but you do not have to start with 'perfect'. Just start.

I really encourage people to do thirty minutes, three times a week as a starting point if you can commit to that, and then build up from there. It might even be, that you can only exercise once this week. In that case, just do once. If you can commit to twice, do twice. The important thing is to start somewhere. That's what people underestimate. People say, "well I can't do three times a week" or "I can't do four times a week this week, so there's no point". In that case, just start doing once in the first week. Once is better than zero, and twice is better than once, three times is better than twice. It's making that commitment to do something once, to get started and then you can build from there.

I'm a big believer in HIIT, which is High Intensity Interval Training. It's good for many reasons. Firstly, it's quick. You can do a good workout in twenty minutes. The extra ten minutes can be used for warming up, cooling down and stretching. It's effective because with body weight HIIT it's a combination of cardiovascular exercise and resistance, for a combination of both types of training. You're getting some resistance training and some cardiovascular training at the same time and it will only take a tiny amount of time out of your day.

Anyone can do HIIT, and you can do it anywhere. You can do it in the smallest of spaces and work at your maximum effort, which means it can scale up or down as far as you need it to. Whatever your maximum effort is, that's where you start, and you improve on that. My maximum is different from your maximum effort, which is again different from anybody else's. You can see improvements very quickly with this kind of training.

One of my clients started doing press ups on her knees at the beginning and she now does ten press ups on her toes. When she started she couldn't possibly do that, but she got stronger and lighter over time and very quickly is capable of much more than she thought possible before.

Finally, you can do HIIT anywhere. You can do it if you're traveling in a small hotel room, at home, at your mate's house, outside, you really can do it anywhere. You just need a small amount of space, enough room for the size of your body. If you want specific instruction on how to do these workouts you can go to www.lisaalicoach.com/workout and follow my workout programme.

Sometimes I just do sprints on the spot. Doing maximum effort work for thirty seconds, and then recovering for a minute. It's a two to one ratio of rest to work. You can do fifteen seconds maximum work, and thirty seconds recovery. You can do thirty seconds work with a minute recovery, or one-minute work and two minutes of recovery. The beauty is you can do that with sprints on the spot. Usain Bolt on the spot; high knees and arms pumping, you don't even have to know what you're doing. Just work hard. Get a timer and go. Start running on the spot. You're going to elevate your heart rate and burn calories, just by moving. It doesn't have to be more complicated than that.

If you're not comfortable or confident exercising, simply look at what you like doing. Do you like dance class? Do you like swimming? Start there and build your confidence.

I should say at this point that if you have any injuries, or you're unsure, always chat with your doctor first, before you start any exercise plan, to make sure you know what your limitations are. Mostly we know what our limitations are but check to be safe.

I've worked with people who have long-term conditions, things ranging from diabetes, high blood pressure through to real high-end heart conditions, multiple sclerosis, Parkinson's, arthritis, fibromyalgia. All these people used to come into the gym and exercise, but they worked within their limitations. If they were having a flare up of pain, they didn't work out. It's just figuring out what you can do. What's your range of movement? How hard can you push? You can always find something that you can do. Something is always better than doing nothing.

### Action Step

1. Decide what you love doing— Davina DVD, Zumba, walking, whatever it is!

2. Look realistically at how many times you could make a commitment in the coming week— is it once a week? Twice?

3. Write in your diary when you are going to do that exercise session— it makes you more accountable to yourself!

### Lift Weights

Bearing in mind everything that we've talked about and that this isn't the most important question to begin with— what is the best exercise to lose weight?

The best exercise for weight loss is resistance training, or weight training. Cardiovascular exercise is important, and we shouldn't underestimate the benefit of it for our overall health; our hearts, blood pressure and all those sorts of things. However, the best exercise to lose weight is lifting weights.

Lifting weights will also help to tone your body. Most people say to me, "I don't just want to lose weight. I want to tone up too". If you want to tone up, you need to do some form of weight bearing exercise. You can start with bodyweight exercises; things like squats, lunges, press ups, planks, etc. We combine a lot of these exercises in the HIIT workouts that I do.

Doing weight bearing exercise will give you the shape that you want and help you to burn fat and get slimmer quicker. This is because the more lean muscle tissue you have on your body, the more fat you will be burning. Having more muscle mass increases your BMR as mentioned earlier. This means you will be burning more calories all the time, just to sustain your body.

I want to dispel a big myth— that lifting weights makes you bulky. This is just not true. The women you see who have large, developed muscles have worked exceptionally hard to look like this over a period of many years. They are likely to be squatting and leg pressing one-and-a-half to two times their own body weight. They are also likely to be eating a very strict diet with specific timings. Genetically, women have less testosterone than men and will struggle to gain that size and bulk. It doesn't happen by accident, and it certainly doesn't happen overnight.

A lot of people wonder whether they must exercise each body part separately. A great way to do weights, which is fun, is to go to something like a circuit training class, or a class like body pump; where the instructor will show you what to do. This will give you a full body weights-based workout, under the watchful eye of a professional. You can build up your confidence and use the support of a class structure while you get comfortable with weights-based training.

If you're on your own and go into any gym, you can always ask for help. There will be gym instructors who can help you put a programme together. However, if you don't like going to the gym, or training with other people, you can do body weight exercises at home. You can get some resistance bands and use them to workout at home.

Download my home or hotel workout programme at www.LisaAliCoach.com/home-workout.

My client Amanda says, "when I first started working with Lisa, she just encouraged me to walk the dog more". Amanda went on YouTube and started following some HIIT workouts on her own after previously saying that she would never go to the gym.

She didn't want to go to the gym initially because she'd had bad experiences in the past, but as her confidence built up, and her body shape changed, she started saying, "you know, I need to go to the gym to shape my body", and she began going on her own. Now she was in a position that she relished the challenge of overcoming her boundaries.

She used to go swimming a lot and enjoyed it. We worked out when she could go swimming again. She would plan it in her diary to go after she dropped her daughter at school. She'd go straight to the baths and swim in the mornings. The more she did it, the more confident she became. The more that she saw the changes in her body shape, the more she wanted to work out. In the end, and completely her own choice, she joined the gym. She realized that she loved it once she'd got in the headspace to go there with the goal of improving herself.

Amanda found a combination of doing things that she loved. She still did her dog walking, still swimming and then she started incorporating some weight training into her programme. Of course, this all started to dramatically change her body shape and combined with the work we did on her diet, she was very successful in her weight loss.

Another client, Ned, was an avid runner. She'd always been a runner and when we began working together she started incorporating bodyweight exercises and HIIT training into her routine. It changed her shape rapidly. When you can see your shape changing, that encourages you, it gives you the belief and the confidence to keep going. You need to see yourself changing, to see exactly what is going on. To be able to visually point a finger at the progress you are making. I always encourage people to take pictures of themselves. Then they can see their shape changing by looking back and comparing the photos against each other.

When taking photos of yourself, it doesn't matter how you take them so much, but that you do them consistently. You need to be able to compare them against each other, side by side. You can take them in a full-length mirror as a selfie— stand in the same spot, on the same day, at the same time— take one each from the front, side, and back. If you don't have a full-length mirror you can ask someone else to take them for you. Just make sure you and they are stood in the same place each time. You can wear shorts, a bikini, or something where you can see your shape. No baggy jumpers!

My client Paula was relatively active, she had some DVD's she used to follow a couple of times per week. As we progressed through the programme she started to bring in some extra activity with NEAT. By the end of the programme she's now going to the gym three times per week and loves it. She told me that her old programme had become too easy and she preferred the gym now.

Your confidence grows by doing things that you enjoy, losing some of the weight, and starting to change your shape. When you have this momentum, you start to see the opportunities for expanding out into doing new things and different things, to push your boundaries and achieve even more success.

## Exercise Recap

Just do more. If right now you walk once a week, start to walk twice a week. If you like swimming, go swimming once a week. Book a Zumba class if that's what you're into. This won't give you the body of a supermodel, of course. What it will do is get you started burning more calories and losing a few pounds.

Is it easy to start with something that you're comfortable with? Yes. It's easier than trying to do something new, or something you don't like. Will it make a difference in your shape and weight? Yes. The government recommends you do 10,000 steps a day. There's a reason they say that. It does make a difference. Exercise doesn't have to be complicated or miserable.

Can you commit to thirty minutes, three times a week? Can you commit to thirty minutes twice a week? Can you commit thirty minutes once a week?

Everyone can at the very least commit to thirty minutes once a week. Make the commitment that you know you can keep. If that's once a week, thirty minutes, twice a week, or three times-a week for thirty minutes, just make that commitment to yourself and diarise it. Look through your diary now and find the time where you can make that commitment and put it in your schedule.

If you say you can't commit to once a week, for thirty minutes, I would question whether that is true or not? We can always find thirty minutes in our week. When we say we cannot find time, it is usually indicative of something else; like you don't like exercise, or you don't feel comfortable doing it. That's totally fine, and there is no judgement on that, but be honest with yourself about the reasons.

I was always a regular exerciser. That wasn't my issue, I didn't struggle getting into the gym three or four times a week. You might find that you're surprised at what you enjoy, once you get into it. I never thought I would like weight training. I thought it was something that other people did; it was for other people, but not for me. When I saw how it can change my shape and how it made me feel strong— feeling strong, rather than just skinny— I started to love it. Strong is the new skinny, as they say. Now I can't imagine not doing weights when I go to my gym in Spain. They're all like, "oh try this, gravity class", or something. I have zero interest. I just like doing weights. It's what I do now.

If you give something a go you might be surprised at what you enjoy. For example, maybe you're working away from home. There's a gym close to the office. You see that it's got a class running and you like the sound of it. Why not give it a try? We're creatures of habit, we don't particularly like to change, but there is a good chance that you'll be surprised at what you like if you do make the commitment to trying new things.

Some people get embarrassed about going into the gym because they think people are looking at them. I can tell you, the chances are they're not. People are much more interested in themselves than they are anybody else!

A potential client once said to me, "I don't want to go swimming with my grandchildren because I think people will be looking at me in my swimming costume. I think they're judging me". That's a very real perception that a lot of people have. It's how this woman *felt*. In truth, the reality is that most people are probably judging themselves in their swimming costumes, and have not got the time, the energy, or the effort to be looking at other people and judging them.

It's the same when you go into the weights room, you think everyone's going to be looking at you in the weights room. I remember one client saying, "I went in there and I thought, people are going to be looking at me and wondering what I'm doing?". She went on to say, "Once I started, I realized nobody actually cares. They're all doing their own thing". Just focus on yourself and suspend worrying about everyone else.

## Action Steps

1. Think what you like to do. It might be Zumba class, an exercise DVD, or jogging around the park.

2. Find 30 minutes in your diary 1-3 times per week and commit to doing this exercise.

3. Move more in your general life. Walk, take the stairs, weed the garden; do anything that burns a few extra calories.

# 4 LIFESTYLE

We began this book by talking about the simple equation for weight loss, which is the same for everybody. The basic calories in versus calories out formula for weight loss. Everybody is the same in this sense, we all lose weight in the same way, but what is different from person to person is that everybody has a unique lifestyle. *How* we do things might be different, even though what we do will be the same.

A lot of the people I work with work away from home; the dual life of living half of the time in a hotel and half at home. Some people have family commitments, young children, or elderly relatives that need caring for. Each situation is unique. Diet clubs and other solutions don't even take this into account. If you can't go to a meeting or follow the plan, you just lose your money. They won't take into consideration that you might be working a ten-hour day or live a very active lifestyle.

With my clients we look at the two- three changes each week that they can implement. It's important that we make a commitment and stick to that commitment. It might be that they're travelling and can't go to the gym three times that week, so we may look at them doing a hotel workout. Maybe they have three meals out in one week, so we focus on breakfast and lunch, and ensure they're getting those two good meals each day. Then they have a little more flexibility to enjoy those meals out, without feeling like it has ruined their diet.

The difficulty with a traditional diet is that you think you've failed if you don't do everything perfectly. It's not about being perfect. The truth is, you will never be perfect. It's about taking imperfect action, irrespective of your lifestyle. Commit to doing what you can, do it consistently, and you will see results.

## How To Create Easy Routines

I had a client who has really struggled previously with her weight. She gets a bit of traction and then stops herself. She was drinking plenty of water each day for a while, and then stopped for no clear reason that she was aware of.

It's about choice and control. When I used to get up and go to work in an office, I had a choice when the alarm went off; I could either get up, or not. The choice was if I get up and go to work it equals me getting paid. If I don't go, I don't get paid and the boss probably won't be very happy. You can brush your teeth and have nice white pearlies, or don't brush your teeth, have bad breath and rotten teeth. It's a choice. We just don't see these choices as negotiable.

When you start to make these choices, it becomes routine. You don't even think about it. The alarm goes off, and maybe it's a bit of a struggle, but you don't really think, "I'm not going to work today", because it's part of a routine. Likewise, you wouldn't say, "I'm not going to bother to brush my teeth today".

Everything you do repeatedly becomes a habit. You create habits by going and immediately putting the kettle on when you come downstairs to make a cup of coffee. The question to ask yourself is how could we apply this to our health and fitness? Creating habits and routines that benefit us and help us reach our goals.

People talk about different amounts of time it takes to create a habit. From 21 days up to 60 days. The research is mixed, but to be on the safe side I assume it's probably a bit longer than that. My transformation programme is twelve weeks long, because it is based on changing your habits for long-term success. It's not just losing weight this month but putting the habits in place to permanently create change.

Another client previously said to me, "I want to be like one of those really successful entrepreneurs like Bill Gates". I asked what she meant, and she said, "you know, somebody who's just really successful and has plenty of time to exercise, is healthy, has a great business and makes loads of money". Truth is, that didn't just come. You must do things to make that happen.

You must create routines and habits to achieve what you want and be able to do what you want with your time. Willpower alone, in my opinion, won't get you there. You must change your habits and routines so that it happens by default, without effort.

Start by picking things you want to change and making it part of a new routine.

Here's a simple checklist of habits to consider.

- Eat 5 portions of fruit and vegetables a day.
- Drink 2 litres of water a day.
- Exercise moderately 3x a week for 30 minutes.
- Sleep 7-9 hours every night.
- Eat a quality piece of protein with every meal.
- Make time for yourself to recharge your batteries and relax each day.
- Eat less than 7 processed meals or meals out per week.
- Drink alcohol less than 3 evenings a week/14 units per week.
- Eat high quality carbohydrates daily.
- Eat good fats daily.

When you want to make changes to your lifestyle the first important part is to break it down into smaller steps— into bite-sized chunks

Overwhelm is the reason people fail on diets. It's simply too much, too fast. When you try and overhaul your entire life, it's completely alien to you. How are you ever supposed to change everything you do in one go?

You can make it so that every day it is a small challenge. Start with, "when I put the kettle on in the morning to make my tea or coffee, I'm going to drink a glass of water, because I know I don't drink enough water". Do that and you are making progress. You're better off than you were yesterday. If you do that often enough, it's just part of your routine. It becomes a habit. Now it will happen every day, without you needing to think about it.

Success comes from breaking things down and taking action. You can focus on those inputs, rather than the outcome. We all tend to say, "I want to lose two pounds," or "I went for my weigh in and I lost three pounds this week".

The focus on the outcome is very natural. That is why we are doing this in the first place, after all. However, if you can detach yourself from the outcome, and instead focus on the inputs; focus on drinking more water, eating more protein, eating more fruits and vegetables; breaking down the process you need to go through to build the habits that lead to weight loss; you get more traction and the outcome will look after itself. Take action, focus on the inputs and then when the weight loss starts to happen, the motivation will follow.

Even if you don't have a stable routine - perhaps you travel for work, or have an unpredictable family situation, you can still pre-plan and not leave things up to chance. If your routine is not stable, say for example, if you're working away from home, you can still choose to take back control.

Supposing you work away four days in the week. On a Monday you must get up and go away in the morning. You do the Sunday night bag pack; have your stuff ready and get on that train or get in the car at X time in the morning. That is a routine. We all have a routine, even if it's not as structured as some people's, we still have a routine. It's a question of how we fit things in around that routine.

When you do the Sunday night bag pack, do you also make your breakfast for the next day, so you can have something that serves your goals? I used to make things like hard boiled eggs, some tomatoes, and lean meat. I would eat it in a traffic jam on the M25 with my cup of coffee. I didn't get into the office having been up however many hours feeling ravenous, waiting until somebody says, "I've brought my leftover cake in", and inevitably end up eating it. How could you resist when you're starving?

You can still create routines, it's about playing the cards you're dealt. Focus on pre-planning, rather than leaving it to chance. Even the most chaotic of routines is something you can make the best of should you choose. Through our work, especially project planners and people like that, we are used to doing this. It is part of our job.

A lot of people say, "I can manage projects at work, but I can't manage my life". It simply requires a little bit of focus and planning. It's obviously not that people don't have the capacity for it. At work they do it successfully. They just don't prioritise it for their health and lifestyle. I think it comes back to people thinking things must be fancy and complicated to be successful, rather than taking those small steps to move forwards.

An example of a small step might be saying, "I'm going to make sure I've got my breakfast in the car or on the train with me. I can do it the night before when I'm cooking my dinner". Instead of thinking, "I've got to have this fancy breakfast and do all these difficult things".

Or people think, "I can't do it, if I'm only going to do ten minutes of exercise when I get up in the morning that's going to be meaningless". They think there's not going to be value in doing it. That is just not the case. Doing something is always better than doing nothing. Do not overcomplicate this.

With that "just do a bit more" attitude, you start to get traction. I think for people that I work with there's probably a little bit of a sense of embarrassment. "I'm very successful in my career but struggling in this part of my life". A lot of people say, "I know what to do. I just need to do it". That might well be the case, but if you don't know *how* to do it, you still need some help.

With action comes motivation as we start to feel better and see results. With motivation comes confidence that we can make a difference. With that confidence and motivation come the results. Once you see results, your mindset starts to change positively, and with this habits become ingrained. I call it my "cycle of success". Remember, action comes before motivation.

## Prioritising The Big Rocks

People think its selfish, women particularly, to take the time and energy to do something for themselves. Especially if you've got children and there just isn't much time in the day to do things solely for yourself. That's why it is so important to place focus on creating these easy routines. You can create the time instead of having to find it in a busy schedule.

Lots of people say to me, "I phone fiddle far too much". People know their own weaknesses, but they often don't know what to do to make positive changes. They don't know how to start. Clients say, "I know what I should do, but I don't necessarily know how to do it". Applying some of those work skills to yourself will hold you in good stead.

You wouldn't just sit down at your desk and say, "I'm going to finish the project today". No— it's planned out. It's time-lined. It's broken down into tasks. You can't complete one bit until you've done the previous bit. It's about breaking your health and fitness routine down to those smaller chunks. Looking at where you could find, or make, the time. Could you find thirty minutes, three times a week, where you can do something? Can you start with just one exercise session of thirty minutes each week?

Can you start by making sure that you drink more water? You have a glass of water when you put the kettle on in the morning, or you put post-it notes on your computer screen saying, "drink more water!", to remind yourself. Get a half litre bottle and fill it up twice. Leave it on your desk so it's there in front of you for easy access, and as a reminder. It's the simple stuff that gets you started, builds momentum and starts to bring results.

People think simple isn't going to work. I thought like that when I first began. When I started with my coach Tim, I wanted to change everything on day one. He said, "stop worrying about protein powder when you're drinking four or five nights a week, consuming a bottle of white each night". People think you've got to have this complexity and the 'perfect plan', but you don't. You can start, have a good breakfast with some protein and fats in it, and drink more water. Go from there.

For some of us, its often a case of, "I'll grab a bit of toast in the canteen" or "I'll just have a bowl of cereal", "I'll get one of those tubs of porridge". They think they're being healthy doing that. You would be better off getting a couple of boiled eggs and some spinach.

After that, start with one thing you can do with exercise and one thing around your lifestyle. Maybe that's drink more water or make sure you switch your phone off at a certain time of night, so you get a good night's sleep.

Then it's one more thing around your food. Perhaps it's to be consciously aware of what you're eating. Do your food diaries and keep track of what is going on to raise your awareness.

Eat, sleep, rinse, repeat. Just do it again the next day. Drink the water, walk the 10 minutes. Do it the same again the next day, and the next day after that. Just do it. You have enough time, it's about priorities and making it fit into your routine, instead of looking at why it won't fit. Once you've done it day after day for a while, it becomes habitual. Then you can layer more new habits in. Soon, you've made significant changes to your lifestyle, but it never felt overwhelming because you did just 2-3 things at a time.

## Being Selfish To Succeed

To see the success you're looking for, you need to make your body transformation a priority. You need to make yourself a priority. So many people have said to me, "I'm at the bottom of the long list of priorities".

Are you going to say that when you're dead and buried? You've burnt yourself out, haven't looked after yourself, you haven't put any care into yourself. You've got to ask how much do you value yourself? The kids come first, yes, and when you're dead who's going to look after them?

What I want to get across is that it's not selfish to take care of your body. You've only got one body, you've only got the one life. Why is it selfish that you should be as fit and healthy as you possibly can? When you are fit and healthy, your energy breeds more energy, and confidence breeds more confidence. When you take responsibility and look after yourself, you have a lot more capacity for everybody else around you.

It's not selfish for example, to ask somebody to look after the kids so you can go to the gym. That might be difficult, but it's certainly not selfish. It's not selfish to say, "I don't want to go out tonight because I don't want to drink". It's not selfish to say, "do you mind if we go to this healthy restaurant rather than the pizza place, because I can get a healthier choice of meal that fits my diet".

One of my clients, Jane's partner works away. When he comes home he always buys her a Danish. I call him Danish Dave. She doesn't really like them, she just eats them because she doesn't want to upset him. He's being kind and thoughtful, and she doesn't want to say that she doesn't want it. I asked why didn't she tell him?

"If you don't want him to buy them, just have a word with him. What's he going to say?". He won't sit her down and force a Danish down her throat. When she did talk to him of course he was very supportive and said he wasn't going to buy them anymore. He totally understood. She'd been doing something that wasn't benefitting her, to try and please someone else, who didn't even care about it. He was totally fine with her refusing.

What's the worst that can happen if you choose to do something for yourself? I always say, start from, "what's the worst-case scenario?".

What if I can't make a living from fitness, what am I going to do? What's the worst-case scenario? For me, I would always say, "I can type really quickly. I could always get transcribing work. I could always have gone and been a PA". That was my background years ago. I could have always got work somehow.

Worst case scenario, I'll give myself this amount of time. If it really gets bad, I'll go and work in a pub because I've done bar work before. If it got even worse, I'll have to go and clean. If I needed money for the mortgage, would I take a job as a cleaner? Yeah. Of course, that worst case scenario never actually happened. It rarely ever will. Regardless, it's freeing to admit what is the worst that could possibly happen.

What would be the worst that could happen if you turn around and said to your husband, "could we go to this restaurant instead? Not that one, not the pizza place, because I want to have a healthier meal". What's he going to say? What's the worst thing he could say? What would your reaction be? It's a case of adjusting those fears to being realistic.

I think there's also a control thing for a lot of women. "Nobody can do it like I do it". We don't let things go, always thinking that we're in a much better place to do it than anyone else in our lives.

This can hold us back and stop us from doing what we really want, because we're so busy trying to control everything and everyone else that we don't have the time or head space to do something for ourselves.

Getting fitter and healthier needs less time than you think. You don't have to battle your way on the treadmill and spend an hour or more plodding away to get results. You don't have to cook fancy food or different foods, you don't need fancy diet meals to get results. Keep things simple.

I used to do double up cooking. When I was making my dinner in the evening, I would make my breakfast and lunch at the same time. It wasn't taking me extra time, it was all done at the same time. Now I could eat the same healthy food at every meal, instead of picking up something to take away for lunch at the office.

If you're in a hotel that has breakfast, why not bring a bit of tinfoil and do a pack-up on the way out from the breakfast bar? When I was in Spain a couple of years ago I was doing a fitness competition, I was so creative with keeping to my diet it was unbelievable. I would go into breakfast, bring my own porridge oats in a bag, I'd get hot water and some of my toffee drops (flavouring). I'd go and get my yogurt and put it in a tub with some pineapple, so I could have that before my workout. Then I'd ask for hard boiled eggs. I'd ask for 4; eat a couple and take a couple with me for later. I was simply taking control of the situation and doing what I needed to do to get the results I wanted.

It doesn't have to take extra time— if you're going into the office in the morning, spend five minutes to stop before you go in and pick up your lunch. Then you're not in a rush. You don't end up justifying eating fast food, "I've run out of time, I had a meeting. I'll just grab a pastry".

All offices have a fridge. Stick some food in the fridge for later. It doesn't have to take more time to eat healthily, it's just a question of being clever with the time that you have and giving it some conscious effort, to make it a priority and make the right choices.

## The More You Do It, The Easier It Becomes

Success comes from creating these positive habits. To begin, it takes a little bit of a thought process. Like my client Ned says, "you have to take a certain amount of responsibility for yourself. You must understand that nobody else can do it for you, but equally, once you start doing it, it becomes routine. It becomes easier. You form habits. Particularly when you see the results and get lots of positive reinforcement".

Action comes first, then results, then motivation. I think that's what people really underestimate, how it spurs you on when you see the results. You want to do more when you're seeing success. People don't believe that because they don't know where to start and are not used to seeing great results without having to upheave their whole life on some unsustainable plan. Give it a go, see success, and I promise you will be more motivated than ever.

When you're on an airplane and they tell you in the event of an emergency to fix your oxygen mask first before helping others, would you say, "no I'm not going to do that", or would you just do it?

They tell you that because if somebody is less able to do it, you will be better positioned to help them by putting yourself first and taking responsibility for yourself, before you worry about them. You will be able to help minors or disabled people or anybody that can't do it themselves only after you have sorted your own wellbeing out. If you try to help everyone else first *you* will be the one who passes out. Then they will be left on their own anyway.

I bring this up because a lot of people struggle to say "no" to things. By saying no, you're not being rude, it's just taking responsibility for yourself first. There's a difference between being assertive and being rude. It's fine to take responsibility for yourself and say no to things when you need to.

I called a client of mine once. It wasn't our regular time to speak, but I wanted to ask her about something. She said to me, "I'm just about to go out, Lisa". I said it was not a problem and asked if she was around later that night? She asked, "is it going to take long?". I said about fifteen to twenty minutes to have a quick chat about something. She said she was going to be late back. I told her not to worry about it and we can speak tomorrow, if she has time. "Yeah, that's not a problem. I can speak to you tomorrow".

When I spoke to her the following day she told me that she never says no to people and mentioned how empowered she felt saying no to talking to me. I told her that I didn't even feel that she had said no to me. I just thought "she's going out the door, that's perfectly reasonable. She hasn't got time to speak to me". Whereas she felt completely overwhelmed that she had been able to say, "I can't talk to you right now. That's not possible".

It's often just small things like this, that other people don't even notice, that can start to build your confidence. I wasn't thinking, "Oh my God, she didn't want to talk to me". It wasn't an issue in the slightest. Putting yourself first is perfectly acceptable.

I was talking to a woman recently who was desperate to have a baby. She had saved all this money to keep having IVF treatment. She has a full-time job and runs three online Facebook groups. She said she doesn't say no to her boss. Whenever her boss says, "can you take this on? Can you take that on?", she never says no. She always takes it on, even when she knows that she shouldn't. When she knows she hasn't got the capacity and is already overwhelmed, she still doesn't say no.

I used to simply say, "no, I can't". People would be shocked that I was professionally assertive, that I would say, "no". Of course, I would always qualify it. When they would look gob smacked I'd say, "well, I can but what do you want me to give up? Because if I take this on, I haven't got time to do this other thing, and that is a priority because...".

This is a problem for a lot of women, particularly when you are competent at what you do. You get assigned that "Lisa can do it because she can do everything" thought by people. The reality is, no, I can't do everything at once.

Being able to say no came from years of being self-employed as an interim and years of saying, "No. That's not what I'm here to do. I want to help, I want to do a good job, but actually I can't take that on because I haven't got enough hours in the day". Saying no is a skill. It is not being selfish but allowing you to fulfil the commitments you already have to the best of your ability. If you spread yourself too thin, nothing gets done and everyone is left disappointed.

It's about asking what's important to you? It was never important to me to be liked at work. I wasn't paid to be liked. I was paid to do a good job. At the end of the day, I was liked because I was so totally, brutally honest. People loved that honesty in me. Instead of trying to appease other people, wouldn't it be better that you liked yourself more? Instead of catering to everyone else to your own detriment, wouldn't it be better to do what is right for you?

It's baby steps. I'm not saying for one minute that you go in and tell your boss to piss off. It's baby steps to being more assertive in a professional and friendly manner.

I was talking to a woman the other day who said, "he's just given me something else to do". This is after I said to her that I didn't think she would be a good fit to work with me on my programme. I asked if she had considered asking to do job share or reduce her hours? She said that was a good idea. She wanted to be self-employed, ultimately. I told her it sounds like your boss values you. Why don't you have the conversation? Just have the conversation. What's the worst that could happen?

As I said, being assertive doesn't mean being rude. It's just doing those little things to create boundaries for yourself. You can start by saying, "can I check because I have got these other things on and I don't want to commit to something that I can't actually do". Instead of just saying, "Yes, I'll do it". Even just taking that step back and saying, "can I just double check before I make that commitment?" is progress and puts you back in control.

Are you somebody that when your friend says, "do you want to meet for a drink tonight?", you still say yes, even if you're tired and would prefer not to? What could you say instead? You might think that you couldn't really say no. Whereas, I'd just say, "could we do it another night? Can I ring you? I'm just knackered tonight". There are ways in which you can manage your own life, without damaging relationships with anybody else.

## Age Is Not A Barrier

I've had lots of people say to me, "can you write in your book about health-related conditions, or what to do if you're menopausal?". The first thing I want to say is that it's never too late. Everyone can make changes to their life and there's always hope for a better future.

Don't think, "I'm 50, I can't change". You can change if you decide to do so. I'm not expecting people to be like me, where I did a fitness competition at 53, but there's always hope for positive changes.

Age is just a number. Is it more difficult to lose weight as you get older? For me, losing weight when I was 49 and coming into my 50s was easier than in my 30s. It was much simpler because I had always tried to overcomplicate it in the past. I'd always try to change everything and then I would fail because it was too much to do all at once. It was overwhelming and too far away from what I had been doing previously.

The right plan will work regardless of age. Most of the people I work with are into their 40s and some are in their late 40s, early 50s. If they've done it, then you can do it too.

*If them, why not you?*

One of my clients is 57, has a grown-up son and works a 60-hour work week as a consultant. She's a social worker by trade, so she has a very caring nature. While often traveling, she lost 16 pounds and 26 inches in 12 weeks working with me. In her own words she said, "you put everyone else first, don't you? I have to put myself first for once". That was the realisation that allowed her to finally lose the weight. She made it a priority and committed to doing what was right for herself, first.

Another, into her 50's, has four kids, one with special needs. She has horses and dogs too. I used to call her Wonder Woman because she always had stuff to do, but always handled it. She made small changes to make things more sustainable like we've discussed in this book and she got the results she had been looking for, despite her commitments and busy lifestyle.

*If them, why not you?*

What is different about you? I could put in lots of examples of different people. Victor, he's a guy obviously, but the principles are the same. He lost 12 and a half pounds in 6 weeks. I spoke to him a couple of weeks ago and he's even lower than the goal that we originally set. He's carried on with the good work we started together and continued to see results. He's a Programme Manager, has a very busy life; he was a classic example of someone managing programmes, but couldn't manage himself. The biggest problem was getting him to eat more, surprisingly.

I do have a couple of people that I've worked with, who used to eat 1,100 calories per day regularly. I said you've got to start eating more. One woman was running, running, running like a demon. The truth is, you're not going to lose weight by beating yourself into the ground. This is about your lifestyle. The only difference between those who succeed, and those who stay stuck is how you manage your lifestyle.

That's why I say to people, of course you can go to diet club if you fancy, but it doesn't take your lifestyle into consideration. It doesn't look at you as an individual. It doesn't allow you to say, "I work away from home 5 days a week and then I'm home at the weekends". The diet club won't consider that. You're on your own to try and figure out how to fit the plan into your lifestyle. That is the reality, you're not a robot but a human being with things going on.

You cannot expect to follow the plan if your lifestyle doesn't allow it, but you cannot expect to get results if you don't follow the plan. This is why a bespoke plan that considers your lifestyle is so important.

I used to work with exercise referral clients who have been referred by their GP to work out and had conditions from high blood pressure through diabetes, fibromyalgia, osteoarthritis, heart conditions, people who've had heart attacks. Honestly, I don't know how they do it. Despite having MS, Parkinson's, some of the guys are amazing. They work within their limitations, but they do not give up. They do not believe that their chronic condition is something that should stop them being as fit and healthy as they can be. It's people like this that are inspirational. They've made a choice to do as much as they can, despite their limitations.

I used to work with one awesome woman who was a weight loss client named Sue. She had fibromyalgia. If she had a flare up she might be in bed for 3 weeks. As soon as that flare up reduced she would be back in the gym and immediately she would get back on and do it. If you do have conditions, check with your doctor first. Speak with them and ask whether you are okay to exercise or change your diet before you do anything. Firstly, ask them whether you're okay to go ahead and secondly, find out what specifically you can safely do.

If you're in the UK and you can get an exercise referral programme from your GP, do it. Often, they're heavily subsidised, plus you get specialists who can support you to put together a plan and programme based on your needs while managing your condition. You also get to be around people who are in the same boat as you, which always helps to keep spirits high.

Don't forget there are places where you can get that support if you do have very specific conditions that you're worried about. In Hastings, we've got this friend who's 83 years old. He cycles up from the sea, plays tennis, cycles home, and then goes for a round of golf in the afternoon. Not only is he 83, but he's had a heart triple bypass when he was in his 50's. What is possible for you is simply about the mindset that you bring.

Sometimes my back plays up. When my back is bad I might use the treadmill and do an arms workout, if I can't do legs or anything involving my back. I just won't do anything that hurts. I will do things seated or with lighter weights, or whatever I need to do to make it happen. The key is finding out what you can do and making the best of it. Find what you can do within your limitations and commit to doing that.

Don't see your limitations as an insurmountable barrier. Don't think that having a health issue means you can't do anything. Light, weight-bearing exercise will improve a lot of conditions as well as being good for your general health.

One of my recent clients has spina bifida, which is a condition where the spinal cord is damaged before birth. Weight loss is often more difficult. Of course, losing weight will help reduce the stress on her joints and manage the condition. She has calipers on her legs and has to use a wheelchair, but she still works out. She is an inspiration. She was never successful in her weight loss efforts previously, but with my guidance she lost seventeen pounds— including losing five pounds in one week.

All this despite various flare-ups and other issues. She had a knee injury and asked for a chair-based exercise programme. Going out using her wheelchair, which is a quite a workout pushing your body weight around. She made the decision to do something because she couldn't do her normal exercise, she just did what she could and got the results because of that.

She said, "You took into consideration my condition and lifestyle to find things that I could do". The reality is, she just did it. It wasn't me that made her succeed. She could easily have made excuses about why she couldn't do things, but she didn't. She committed to doing what she could, and it paid off. Here is what she said;

"I have spina bifida, and it's known that people with spina bifida find it difficult to lose weight. I've never been slim, even as a child. A year ago, I got a knee injury that left me wheelchair bound. That meant I couldn't move and do the walking that I used to.

Using a wheelchair for convenience; when you're with people and walking a long way that's one thing— it's a choice. When you haven't got a choice and you're in it all the time, you realise how restrictive it is. How bad for your health it is to be sitting all the time.

That left me fed up. Not quite depressed but you ask yourself, "why bother?". A lot of my clothes were too tight. They didn't look as nice and that made me feel down. I didn't want to go out and buy bigger clothes.

I'd tried all the big dieting clubs that everyone does, and I'd found them to be a one-size fits all, a bit like a robot. You go and pay your money, get weighed and off you go. It's just not personalised enough. It wasn't achieving what I wanted to achieve.

Lisa offered a different approach to anything I'd seen before. She takes the effort to look at you as an individual. Looking at the internal barriers and your motivation. She understood the impact my disability would have on how quickly I could lose weight. Her approach was to change little things—for example drinking more water each day - she didn't ask me to change my way of eating for the first week or so. Just to photograph food and record what I'm eating.

Lisa gave me insight on why I had the eating habits I had. She never told me I couldn't eat anything, just made me aware of what I was doing. Making you aware that you might lose the weight quicker if you choose differently, so the power is always with you to make changes.

I lost just over a stone in twelve weeks, which is amazing because I've done it with less exercise than I've done before when I've lost any weight. I've gone down a clothes size and can't even remember how many inches I've lost. I'm really pleased with the outcome. Having more energy and doing more physical activity, I feel really good. Much happier".

A lot of women say, "I'm peri-menopausal, or menopausal; I can't lose weight". I don't believe that is true. I started my journey at the age of forty-nine and got on stage for a fitness competition at fifty-three, after doing a photoshoot at fifty-two. Was it possible? Yes, I lost weight. At the ages of fifty-two to fifty-three I was the same weight I was in my late teens and early twenties. I was in better shape than I was back then. I had more muscle definition and less body fat.

Was it more difficult? Yes, it was more difficult when I was competing against women who were ten or more years younger than me. Was it harder for me to lose the weight? Yes, it probably was. I don't know for certain because I don't compare myself to other people.

However, the real question is, did I do it? Yes. Was it possible? Yes. Do I still have periods where I think I need to shift a few extra pounds? Yes. All those things are possible.

I'm not underestimating that for some women their hormones can be out of line, and if that is the case you should go to your GP and get checked out. I don't want to underestimate how much the menopause can affect people. I have probably been lucky. I just want to show you what is possible, if you decide to commit to doing it.

It's important to understand that you might have to focus on it a little more. You might have to work a little bit harder. The weight won't fall off you like it might have in your twenties. That isn't just about your hormones, but your metabolism changes, too. Metabolism will slow, muscle mass decreases as we get older, and that is why weight training is so vital, to fight that age-related decline. It helps keep your metabolism higher. The more muscle you have, the more fat you burn, and the better you look. Who wants to be skin and bones? You want to have some tone and definition, which comes from muscle.

I've worked with women of all different ages, many in their forties and fifties. They've all had success, they've all been able to lose weight and keep it off. It might take a little longer to get to where you want to be, but that's ok.

# 5 STRESS AND OVERWHELM

One thing that people really underestimate is how, particularly when you work in jobs where you're an interim, you're only as good as your last contract. Your name is what takes you through. There's a lot of pressure before you even start a job. You don't get the luxury of going in and having inductions. It's, "here, can you go to this meeting in half an hour?". Straight in at the deep end.

I came across somebody again in my last contract that I'd worked with about a decade earlier. My boss had sacked him, and he had cried. Now I came across him ten years later thinking, "I wouldn't employ him", but everyone was raving about him and how good he was. First impressions last and that puts immense pressure on you to always perform at your peak

Then we all have lives around that; at home, relationships, kids, etc. People underestimate how much stress can impact you if you're wanting to lose weight. While we typically understand that stress impacts you in terms of high blood pressure and that sort of thing, not so many people know that it can stop you losing weight.

For long periods, excess stress can raise your cortisol levels (your stress hormone). This can lead to holding on to belly fat. To help lose weight, and free up the time and headspace to do everything else mentioned in this book; managing stress is a key component.

Sleep is an important foundation for effective weight loss, and if you're not sleeping enough then you are adding a massive burden of stress on top of everything else. My client Paula, who I was talking to last week just moved in with her fella. They were all over the place a bit, and when she doesn't get her sleep I can tell she struggles. To get back into a routine and on top of her stress she makes a conscious decision. She puts her phone on airplane mode to make sure she gets seven to nine hours of sleep every night.

If you're only getting five or six hours of sleep per night that's not going to help you with your weight loss efforts. You need to get enough sleep. It's going to help reduce your stress, to build and repair your body. We all go through periods of overwhelm, that's life and it is unavoidable. Sleeping is an essential part of human life, as much as water or oxygen and we need to give it focus.

High stress and lack of sleep leads to overwhelm. I think I'm the classic example of this. I had this conversation with my coach, Tim. He said, "do you know how many times since we've known each other you've said to me something always happens?". I'd be going along happily and then something gets thrown at me. I'm like, "oh shit! I've got to deal with this, now! Oh my God, I've got this really big problem".

Life always happens. Whether it's overwhelm through big things happening, or whether it's lots of small things that all add up. It's always going to be Christmas, holidays, somebody's birthday. There's always stuff going on at work, with friends and family. That's never going to go away, it's how you manage it that's important.

How you manage your weight loss efforts and your overall health and wellbeing when you come to terms with the reality that life is not perfect, and things happen that are outside of your control.

If you want to lose weight you need to stay ahead of potential problems. I have the three strategies around holidays, Christmas, birthdays, parties, etc. to keep you on track. These can be applied during your overwhelming moments, when work is crazy, you're moving house, or something else is causing disruption in your life.

Remember, they are to continue with your diet; to be 80% on your diet and have a bit of 'off time' so you maintain your progress; or to say screw it, let loose and deal with the consequences later.

These are strategies that you can implement. You must make the choice of what is important. Do you care more about your weight loss, or about indulging in a binge? Will you grab a takeaway because you're rushed off your feet and tired, or is there a better option? Don't let things happen to you. It's your choice.

If you say, "screw it, I can't deal with it. I'm not going to worry about it right now", that's absolutely fine. That's your choice. What I do strongly recommend people do, is make a choice that they are going to have fun - but not hurt themselves. Get to a certain point and say, "I've had enough".

Don't keep eating or drinking for the sake of it, when you don't even enjoy it any more. If you're using it as stress management, don't indulge it into a binge.

## Coping Mechanisms

What a lot of people do when they feel overwhelmed or feel like they're not coping is go towards comfort eating or drinking too much alcohol. It's perfectly normal, it's perfectly natural. Some people turn to food, some people turn to alcohol, some people turn to drugs. They're all coping mechanisms.

Ultimately, those things aren't going to hold you in good stead in the longer term. Don't beat yourself up about doing it, but also look at how it might be holding you back across multiple parts of your life.

I recommend being curious about your reaction to a situation. I know if I'm stressed, I want to have a drink. I just want to stick my head in the bottle— I know that about myself. A lot of people know that they're comfort eaters, or they're emotional eaters. They know if things are stressful they just want to go and buy several bars of chocolate, to sit and eat the whole lot in one go— which is fine. There is no judgment here, just honesty about the situation.

Hands up how many people feel great afterwards? People generally don't.

They feel ashamed, they feel guilt, they feel disgusted with themselves. They think, "I'm never going to do that again. I'm never going to touch another drop of alcohol. I'm never going to binge eat chocolate again".

How often does that last?

Chocolate and alcohol, we know they are not good for us. Often, we don't even enjoy it. I think that's the starting point to getting control of your binge eating or drinking; to recognise that you're not going to enjoy this afterwards. Take a step back and be curious about why you're doing it and what happens after you do so.

Equally, be curious about why you didn't hit your goals before. That's a really good place to start. Just ask yourself the question, "what went wrong?"

That alone will make a huge difference. Even if you can stop yourself for just one minute and ask, "why am I going to do this? How will it benefit me? Why is it important for me to do this? Will it make me feel better?", you're going to be acting with so much more awareness.

Whatever happens, own it. If you do go ahead and break your diet, take time off on holiday, etc. own it. Don't feel guilty and disgusted afterwards, just say, "I've done it. What have I learned from it?".

It's not the mistakes we make that are important, it's what we learn from them. We all make mistakes. The big thing is that one binge meal is meaningless in the wider scale of things. If you're doing it repetitively, then it might be time to question yourself, or seek professional help. However, one meal is going to make no difference if you're doing everything else right. Don't make one meal the reason to give up. Really it won't make any difference. Just get back on track.

Of course, this is all good, but it brings up the question of what you should do to cope with stress or overwhelm. I find that exercise really helps. Even if it's just walking. I had an interview once and somebody said, "how do you cope with stress? How do you cope when it all gets on top of you?", I said, "I do confide in a trusted colleague if I have a trusted colleague. Other than that, I go for a walk and that helps to clear my head".

If you're feeling overwhelmed, confide in somebody. Talk to somebody who knows you, who gets you. Admit how you feel. "I'm really feeling overwhelmed. I want to eat everything that moves. I want to go out and drink". Just talk it out with somebody. I think that helps a lot. A problem shared is a problem halved, as they say.

If I exercise, even if it's just to get out and walk for ten minutes to take my mind off stuff, I feel much better. I know a lot of people are very busy and perhaps think they don't have time. If you just get up and move away from the situation, even for five minutes, you'll usually feel better. Just go and walk somewhere.

Make those choices, because at the end of the day you're the only person that can change it. Nobody else can change it for you. You've got to make that decision of how you're going to cope with stress or overwhelm. Are you going to revert to typical coping mechanisms like food and alcohol, or are you going to give something else a shot? Will it damage your weight loss efforts if you're regularly and consistently drinking alcohol or emotionally eating? Yes. I would suggest you start looking at other solutions if you really want to change. Burying your head in the sand doesn't help.

For me, I like to use journaling. It can help you get clarity on what you're thinking. For example, when you're being harsh on yourself, "oh, I only lost a pound…", yes, but you need to ask what did you do? What did you do well? What could you have done better?

I start each call with my clients by asking what went well for them this week? What did they achieve? Was there anything they struggled with? Anything they think they could do better?

By journaling about these things, we can look back and see how far we've progressed. It's very motivational when you're thinking you've had a bad week, to look and see that you've actually done lots of things well. You see that you are making progress on this journey. You didn't put the weight on in one to two weeks and it isn't going to come off in one to two weeks. Journaling is simply recording that journey to see how you're getting on.

I still regularly journal myself. It really helps me gain clarity, nowadays around my business and where I want to get to. It makes me much more aware of what is going on, what I'm struggling with, breaking things down into smaller parts and making a commitment to myself by putting pen to paper.

If you're not sure what is going on, writing the questions mentioned above and then answering them really helps to gain clarity. It doesn't have to be something you do every day. It can simply be used as a tool to reflect, to see what you are achieving, and where you want to get to next. You can't just remember everything, and it helps to look back in the future and see just how far you have come.

Let's identify some typical stress triggers, coping mechanisms, and a better option you could turn to.

Stress triggers include…

- Deadlines.
- Increasing volume of work.
- Changing circumstance (moving home, etc.).
- Relationship problems/breakdown.
- Kids.
- Illness.
- Financial problems.
- Unforeseen challenges.
- Poor sleep.

Coping mechanisms include…

- Alcohol.
- Emotional eating.
- Stopping exercising.
- Trouble sleeping.
- Burying self in work, longer hours.
- Withdrawing into yourself.
- Bottling things up.

Better alternatives include…

- Finding someone you trust who you can talk to.
- Writing things down (I regularly journal).

- Exercising even if it's only a walk.
- If you're drinking, drink more water.
- Being aware of it as a passing phase, you'll come out of it.
- If you can't sleep, writing down in a notepad next to your bed, getting things out of your head.
- Trying to be more in the moment when eating.
- If you're really struggling, get professional help.
- Taking a break.

# 6 MOTIVATION

A lot of people say to me that they just need a kick up the behind. They've lost their mojo. Saying things like "I just need a PT to kick me up the backside", or "I know what I need to do, I just need to get my head around it".

That's ok if you just need to lose a few pounds, but in my experience that is not what will keep you going. It's enough to lose four to five pounds, but when you start talking about double figures, you need something more to keep you motivated. What is going to drive you to keep you going after those first few pounds? To achieve your long-term goals?

Most people don't clearly identify what their goals are, unless its someone like a bride who has a really defined goal. That's a very specific point in time, when all eyes will be on you. It's easy to make a specific goal around the pre-determined date. A lot of people say things like "I'm going on holiday" or "I've got a birthday or wedding I'm going to", but those are external factors. They're not actually why you want to change, or what will keep you going beyond the first couple of weeks.

Identifying why you really want to change might take you a bit out of you comfort zone. Staying with what we know is easier, and we feel safer doing it. That's why change is so difficult, because getting out of our comfort zone to make changes to our lifestyle takes a big commitment. You need lasting motivation to push yourself like that. You need to find something truly meaningful, to give you that lasting motivation.

I spoke to a woman who broke down when we were talking, when she spoke about her father's ill-health. Other people say they just want to be a good example for their children. They can see their children picking up their bad habits and realise that they need to do something about it.

Now the goal is bigger than themselves, it's outside of them and for something (their children) more valuable than themselves (in their own mind). Others talk about how they feel every day, about how desperate they feel in their body, and they don't want to live their life like that any longer.

Most people, when they start a diet, don't think about why they really want to do it. When I first start talking to a client, we talk about why they want to lose weight. Ultimately their goal is not, "I want to lose a few pounds". There's a lot more going on around your health and body impacting you, which maybe you don't articulate.

My client Maddy said, "It's not just about the fact you can't run five miles. It's not just that you can't walk up the stairs. It's so much more than that". It was affecting her confidence to the level that she didn't want to speak up at work. She knew stuff, but she didn't want to say it. This was holding her back in her career and stopping her doing the job as effectively as she could.

In her personal life she said, "Even if I had gone on a date, I would doubt why anybody would still want to date me". It doesn't just affect how you look and feel, it's usually much deeper than that, and people don't think about that. It has a massive effect on your confidence, self-worth, and how you portray yourself to other people.

You need to work out why you really want to do this. For a lot of people, they start talking about their health, but it's usually more than that. When I was overweight, but still a qualified fitness professional, my husband said, "You can't tell me what to do. You don't practice what you preach". He was right. If I'm not doing these things, and putting them into practice, how can I help other people to do them?

My weight was fundamentally impacting my ability and belief in myself to be able to do the job that I really wanted to do. If you don't work out your 'why', you will struggle. Willpower will keep you going a certain distance, but it won't get you all the way there.

I wonder, how many people keep it up after losing the initial few pounds? Unless they go a little bit deeper than that and understand why they really want to do this. That's why I say, write it down, be open with yourself. Write everything down because ultimately, it's not just about your weight. It's much bigger than that. Statistically 95% of people who lose weight put it back on… Be one of the 5%.

## Finding Your Why

If you don't know the answer, just ask yourself a series of questions…

*How do I feel about the way I look?*

*How does this impact my ability to run around with the kids?*

*Do I want to be a role model?*

*Am I holding myself back at work?*

*Am I confident?*

*Am I as confident as I think I am or could be?*

A lot of people say, "Oh yeah, I'm really confident". It's a default reaction, but when they think about it, they know they're not. Not like they used to be.

Keep writing until you've got through all the questions. Even think about it as you would say it to a friend, like you were having a conversation with a friend.

*Why do you want to do this?*

*Why is it important to you?*

*What will change in your life if you do this?*

*What do you feel the impact is, on your life, other than just the physicality of your body?*

Don't worry about feeling like this is self-centered or vain. It's not about vanity, it's not just the aesthetics of it. If you don't know why you want to lose weight, you probably won't get to where you want to be.

It's about being honest with yourself. The honesty of admitting if you have any fears holding you back. Honesty is critical. A lot of the time, we get in our own way and hold ourselves back, because we are scared.

It's very rare that people will come to me and never have tried anything to lose weight before. It's uncommon that people will say, "I'm forty-three and I've just put on weight in the last six months to a year". Most people will have tried to lose weight at some point or another. Maybe lost it, then put it back on. It's not something that's happened recently or overnight. It happens steadily, over years and even decades. Why does weight loss never stick? Why do you end up back where you started?

You need to ask yourself:

*What am I scared of?*

*Am I scared of failing again?*

*Am I scared how things might change if I do get more confident and other things might happen in my life because of this?*

If you really can't think about why you want to lose weight, think about the other side of it.

*What would be different if you were your ideal size and shape?*

*How will you feel being able to go into your favourite clothes shop and pick up the size that you want to wear, knowing that it will fit you?*

*How will it feel to be able to go on holiday and know that you can wear a swim suit, and you will feel happy wearing it?*

*How will it feel to be able to have the same energy levels that you have at 9 o'clock in the morning, right through until 6 o'clock in the evening?*

*How will it feel to throw out the fat clothes and open the thin clothes wardrobe?*

*How will it feel to look in the mirror and like what you see, to be happy with yourself?*

*What's your ultimate goal?*

It might be that you say, "I want to lose three stone". When you know your ultimate goal, you can work backwards from there. Most people won't necessarily know how much they want to lose, or how long it will take. It's a case of saying to yourself, "This is where I want to be in the end. Now I'm going to work backwards to break it down in to stages until I get to what I need to do right now".

You want to have that bigger picture. Your first smaller goal might be, "I want to lose seven pounds in four weeks". Or it might be an even smaller goal than that. Something like, "I want to start this week. Even if I only lost a pound, I'd be happy".

There is an amount of self-management involved. You must take responsibility for yourself. Whilst I can say, "you're not drinking enough water", only you can drink more water.

You take responsibility at work. This is exactly what you do at work, all you need to do is do the same thing for yourself. Particularly when you work on projects. You'll accept your work package, and you know what you've got to do, or you know that you've got to deliver something within a certain timeline. You just do it, it's part of the process of working on a project. You need to do the same thing for your health and weight loss. Accept responsibility by recognising that nobody else can do it for you. It's a commitment to taking a level of care for yourself.

I got to a certain point, and you might be here too, where you've put your head in the sand for so long and you don't really care about yourself. I think that's partly fear, because you may have failed many times before. It's easier not to address it, rather than to fail again. The liberating thing is, taking responsibility feels so much better.

Once you get your head out of the sand, and you say, "I've got to do this for me, and nobody else, and I'm going to make that choice and take responsibility", it's liberating. Now you're in control.

I was talking to you previously about willpower versus choice. You choose to get up when the alarm goes off and go to work. You don't have to, but you know that you might get the sack if you don't. You can turn over and go back to sleep. You don't have to get up, but you make that choice. Why not choose to treat yourself kindly and with respect, to look after your body? You know what happens if you don't. Why is lacking self-confidence, lacking energy, ill-health, more acceptable than getting sacked?

Now you have your big goal, and your bite-sized short-term goals to move towards. When I was losing weight, I broke it down in to smaller time scales and chunks of weight loss. I like to do that; it keeps it motivating in the short term, while still having an eye on the long term.

It might be, "I want to lose a pound this week". That could be a short-term goal, and then a medium-term goal might be seven pounds in four weeks.

## Action Steps

1. Get a piece of paper and write down your 'why' as explained above.

2. Keep that close by to remind you of all the positive reasons you started this journey.

3. Be patient. Remember that you didn't gain the weight in a week.

4. Focus on the small inputs; the outcome will take care of itself.

## How To Be In The Right Mindset To Lose Weight

It's curious how people often say to me that they're just not in the right mindset or not motivated to lose weight. They can't seem to start their weight loss journey.

Try this; flip it around. If you just start your journey, that is when your mindset and your motivation will change. If you take action and do one little thing, you feel that you're taking back control. It feels good to say that you've gone to the gym this week when you haven't been for a long time.

When you start making those small changes, your motivation comes back. As you start losing the pounds and inches, that's when your motivation becomes greater. You don't need high motivation to start, you need to take action and the motivation will follow.

Remember the cycle of success is:

- Action.
- Motivation.
- Confidence and success.
- Mindset.
- Habits.

## Project You: Cycle of Success

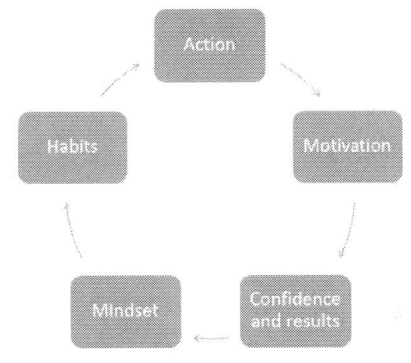

```
        Action
       ↗      ↘
   Habits    Motivation
     ↑          ↓
   Mindset ← Confidence
             and results
```

I talk a lot about taking imperfect action. People think if they can't get to the gym five times this week, or they're going out for drinks this weekend, then there's no point starting a diet until they can get a clear run at it. That's just not so. You don't need to do everything perfectly, every single day. You just need to take that imperfect action and get started. Giving it your best shot and getting on with it.

If you have birthday drinks, or meals out, that's only a couple of things per week. There are twenty-one meals per week that you can do the right things most of the time and one to two meals off shouldn't make a big difference.

What are you committed to doing this week to move towards your goals? Write it down.

## How To Remove Obstacles For Success

There's always something that's going to happen to throw you off track. We need to recognise these obstacles and ask ourselves how we can remove or work around them, before they become something that leads to you struggling or even failing.

I put on ten pounds very quickly when I went back to London to work on my final contract. We had three people in our team that make good cakes, one particularly. She'd make cakes every week and bring them in to the office. I call it the 'office cake culture'. She wouldn't make one cake, she'd make three cakes. It would be like, "this is the Mary Berry lemon drizzle, this is the Starbucks lemon drizzle recipe, and this is my lemon drizzle". You couldn't escape the cakes!

You need to recognise the potential problems. Not say that you can never have a piece of cake, because that's unrealistic, but make your own choice. Not giving in to peer pressure or falling into mindless eating. Maybe you've got those friends that say, "you don't need to lose any weight. You're fine as you are". It's not about anybody else's opinion, it's about what you want to do, and how you feel about it. If you want to lose weight, then that is what you should do.

If you don't want the cake, it's just a case of saying, "no thanks". You don't even have to say that you're on a diet or that you can't eat cake. I just used to say, "no thanks" whenever anybody offered. Soon, people didn't offer me cake any longer. They would just take it for themselves or offer it to someone else because they knew I would turn it down. It wasn't even a thought to offer me it anymore and thus the potential struggle had been removed.

It's recognising the obstacles that might be in your way on a daily basis. A lot of people say, "my husband is like a bloody whippet. He can eat what he wants, and I can't do that". That might be the case. It's important that you're recognising and addressing it, saying, "hey listen, I want to lose weight. I can't eat chips everyday like you do, because that doesn't help me, and I would like your support". Most of the time they will be supportive.

I think most people's potential obstacles will be the same. It might be that you've got certain recurring pinch points. It's late afternoon, the cake comes out, or somebody's brought a packet of biscuits at lunch time. Maybe you're tired and could use a pick me up. This is probably happening on a regular basis. You need to have an alternative. Maybe you get some fruit or nuts and keep them in your desk drawer. I always make sure I've got a healthier snack available. A lot of people find it difficult to say no. That's fine. Instead you want to create an alternative that you can do first, before having to use willpower to say no.

Have a think about the things that you feel are your pinch points. What are they?

Do you say to yourself, "I ate really healthily all day", but when you sit down and think about it, you had two glasses of wine, and then some snacks in the evening? Maybe a sugary coffee in the morning? Only you will know what your pinch points are. The first thing is to identify what they are. Go back to the beginning and look at the food diary and My Fitness Pal data. What does the data tell you? See what is happening and ask *why* that is happening.

Once you've identified your pinch points, make a plan to manage them. There is always a solution; but only after you've identified the problem.

It is likely that you come in, sit down and have a glass of wine without thinking. Try instead to have a glass of water, or say to yourself, "I'll have my glass of wine after dinner instead of before". By then you'll probably not want it.

Sometimes you might struggle when things are not in your control, for example if your partner cooks dinner. It doesn't always have to be a case of eating something different, but maybe you look at the balance and say, "could you make me some extra vegetables?", or you just have a smaller portion. You don't have to change everything, but you do need to address the things that hold you back.

If you don't tell somebody what you're trying to achieve, they won't know to support you. If you haven't said to your partner, "listen, can you help me out. You're doing the dinner, could you just do some extra veg for me?" then you're going to be fighting an unnecessary battle.

It's about you, no one else. Being strong and saying when you don't want something. You've got the cake culture and that isn't going to go away. You can't change that, so you must focus on what you can control, which is yourself. This is about you, it's not about what anyone else thinks. It's your body, it's your life, it's your choice and some people might think that's selfish or annoying, or whatever they want to think. That's their choice. Why is it selfish that you want to lead a healthy life for as long as you can? That's not selfish. That's sensible.

Find yourself a buddy, someone who's got your back. Tell your buddy the truth, "this is really getting me down, I want to lose this weight". If you do, and it's the right person, they'll support you. They won't try and derail you. If it's your partner, and you say, "this is important to me", they should support you. If they say something like, "I love you the way you are", I would say they might love me the way I am, but I don't love myself. Tell them that you want their support.

If you want to go to the pub, you find people who like going to the pub. If you want to get lean, find people who like going to the gym. Spend time with them. Find someone who's invested in their health. Find someone who's going to encourage you to go to the gym. Find someone who doesn't think it's strange that you don't want to eat three slices of cake.

For me, when I was a working at Barnet, my friend Grace and I didn't want to sit eating three slices of cake and drinking skinny tea. We would support each other, bitch about everyone else and say how ridiculous they were thinking skinny tea was going to help lose weight, as they were literally eating cake with the other hand. She took her fitness very seriously, she's a big marathon runner. We used to go to the gym together after work. Having her support really helped to keep me on track. Someone who 'gets it' and is in your corner can be invaluable.

If you don't have access to a fitness buddy in real life, you can get support and accountability online. Come join my group on Facebook. Find a support network. There are plenty of them out there. There are plenty of weight loss groups. You can always find a place where people will support you online. My Facebook group is a non-judgmental, supportive place where you can say what you want. You can ask questions. I'm always posting my best content there first; hints, tips, challenges. You can join us at www.LisaAliCoach.com/group.

Take imperfect action. Have a slice of cake today if you want. That's not going to do you any harm, but it will if you're doing it every day and not accounting for it. If you consistently eat cake, that won't help your weight loss goals, but if you consistently drink lots of water, eat more fruit and veg, that will. Take action, it doesn't have to be perfect, but you do need to get started before you're going to see any results.

As discussed before, just pick one or two things, and focus on changing them for a week. Most people say they don't drink enough water. Make that a goal to focus on for the week. Start by saying, "when I put the kettle on in the morning, I'm going to have a glass of water at the same time. I'm going to buy a little bottle and make sure I drink three of those in the day. I don't eat enough vegetables and fruits so I'm going to make sure I have a portion at every meal".

It takes sixty plus days to create a new habit. You must give yourself a chance to make these new behaviours part of your regular routine. You can do things to make it easy to remember what you're doing like writing what you're going to do in your diary or putting post-it notes on your computer screen. Once you've done it, for one or two days, it will start to become more routine and eventually feels natural.

If you haven't already done it, go back to the questions earlier in this chapter and answer them now. Write down all the cons of what being overweight means to you. How is it affecting you? How do you feel about being overweight? Then write down what will be different if you lost the weight? How will you look and feel at your ideal weight/size/shape?

Be kind to yourself but be honest. It's not about beating yourself up, but you do need to do a bit soul searching to find out and admit how it is impacting you.

# 7 HABITS AND ROUTINES

We've talked about setting goals; aiming for the bigger picture, and then breaking it down. It is best to break it down on a daily and weekly basis. I think it's easiest to make a commitment on a weekly basis and pick one or two things that you focus on each week. Then look at what you need to do each day to meet the weekly goal.

If you're always getting caught out at lunch time, for example maybe you're getting to the office, have a meeting and you haven't got any food to eat so you go to the canteen and there's nothing healthy there. You have to eat something, and you end up with a less healthy option, because it's the only thing that's there. If you're regularly doing that, change that habit. Buy your lunch on the way in. If you know that this is happening to you regularly, get some food in advance. Get some fruit, or whatever fits your diet, before you get to the office. Now you've got your lunch there, you can just grab it whenever and know you've got a healthy choice. Most offices have a kitchen and fridge, so stock up and put extra food in the fridge.

Most of us know where we struggle. It's the same places; drinking more water, never having chance to eat a healthy lunch, grabbing breakfast on the run, struggling to fit going to the gym in as a priority in our schedule.

For breakfast, if you're at home there's no reason you can't get up five minutes earlier to stick some eggs in the microwave and scramble them. It's simply being a little bit creative and focusing on those things you know are a problem for you. Find solutions to those recurring problems and getting results is easy.

I think one of the big things that holds people back is that it doesn't feel like the little effort of making breakfast is going to be enough to see an outcome. It's interesting one of my clients said, "I really thought I didn't have enough time. I never cooked in the evening. I always ordered in, or I got something on the way home. I just didn't think I had enough time to do it myself. I thought it was impossible for me. I didn't think I had enough time to exercise either. It's not that I don't want to, it's just that I haven't got the time. Now, I rarely get take out. I just started doing the things I thought I didn't have time for. The reality was, I did have the time, when I chose to make it a priority".

I think our perception of challenge can be a barrier. When you do it once you realise that you can do it again. Your confidence grows, and then you're able to repeat it. My client said, "actually, I could easily commit to fifteen minutes doing some high intensity interval training (HIIT) at home. I have much more time than I thought I did, when I made it a priority".

She got to this position because we've broken down the journey into manageable chunks. We started with the easier wins. It's not necessarily about tackling the things that you think are most challenging first, but perhaps tackling some of the easier ones.

It might be as simple as, "I'm going to park the car a bit further away and walk for ten minutes". Or it might be, "for my mid-morning snack instead of a biscuit, I'm having an apple or a banana". It's starting with those simpler things. You get momentum and build your confidence to tackle some bigger things later, when you're already seeing results.

Most of my clients identify the problems and recurring issues that they have and rectify them. They know what the obstacles are and start to change them. For example, one of my clients was always grazing on poor food choices. He realised that it didn't take much effort to start making some meals (particularly in the evening) and before long, he found some old recipe books which he went back to in a desire to create better tasting and interesting meals.

Perhaps you can do your meal preparation on Sundays, instead of getting home on Monday night when you're knocked out at 9PM and you're left thinking, "crap, what am I going to eat? I'll have to get takeaway". I've said to people, you can buy packet rice that you put in the microwave, you can buy pre-packed vegetables that you put in a microwave. You can buy pre-cooked meat. It doesn't have to be an enormous task. If you have to stop and think about what to do, because you don't always have something planned or prepared, you are making it more difficult than it needs to be.

Some people ask, "will I have to do a meal plan for the whole week?". No, you don't need to strictly plan out everything, but if you know you're going to be late on Monday, Tuesday, Wednesday then you probably want to know what you're going to have on those evenings. Now you have all the tough times covered and you can catch up again Thursday with some more meal prep, shopping, or just cooking something you enjoy when you have the time and energy spare. A little planning goes a long way in meeting your goals.

One of my clients said she used to mentally check out mid-week. I think that was partly if she hadn't planned what she needed to do, if she was traveling, and perhaps she hadn't taken her lunch with her; she got overwhelmed. So she ended up not doing anything. Falling back into habitual patterns that weren't serving her.

You need a little bit of planning to succeed. I used to say things like that as well. When I went through my own transformation, I changed. If you don't have that little bit of fore planning, it will be harder to reach your goals when you're out and about, when you're busy, when you're tired, or you're stressed.

At work on a project, we wouldn't say, "I should have had a meeting yesterday. Oh well". If we knew that we were on a timeline and there were things we had to do, we'd be prepared and plan it in advance. You don't ask, "what's happening today? I better do something". That would leave you constantly fighting fires. You don't want to be constantly fighting fires in your fitness either.

If you've got action steps from your meeting, you do them before the next meeting. That's what you should do with your fitness too. A lot of people don't do them. It doesn't have to be massive amounts of planning, it can literally be on a day to day basis, if that fits you better, but it's got to be based on what works around your schedule.

If you know, for example, you've got to travel on Wednesday and you've got to be up early, but you normally work out Wednesday morning; you need to plan something. If you know you can't do it, re-plan it for a different time. It's about having a grip on what's going on, each day and taking control of the situation.

When you're going to exercise write it in your diary, make that commitment to yourself, and schedule it. On a Sunday evening, spend ten minutes planning what you've got coming up in the week, and how you can fit your exercise, food preparation, shopping, etc. in around that. If you know, for example, you've got to be up early on Wednesday, and you've got this all-day meeting in a different office. Prepare your food for breakfast that you can take on the train.

To start planning better and taking control you should start with the simplest things. Start with what is the most obvious thing to you. Write down a list of the five most obvious things you know you need to do slightly differently. Create reminders for yourself. Put things in your diary, write notes for yourself, set reminders on your phone.

When you're doing a project, you look at your deadline and work backwards. You'll then put boundaries around it, what resources you need, what time you need to hit the deadline. Do the same thing here. Prioritise your five most obvious things in order, and then create reminders for the most important first.

Change just two- three things per week, to give it time to be cemented into your routines, and to ensure you're not overwhelming yourself with too many things to try and do in one go. If you've worked in the project environment like I did, it's the most natural thing in the world to plan like this, but we often struggle applying it to our daily personal lives. We get overwhelmed and don't know where to start. People think that little things like drinking more water won't make any difference. They don't believe it will make a change, so they don't do it.

If you were planning a project and just sat there and looked at all of it, you'd get overwhelmed and think you couldn't do it. That's why you break it down into tasks, work packages, deliverables, milestones and then you allocate that work. We need to break down our personal lives the same way, into those smaller, more manageable pieces that we can attach specific tasks to.

## Be Action Specific

Most people tell me that they know they don't do "X". Generally, people know where to start, and when someone says that to me, they are usually right.

Identify those areas you know you could look at making improvements in. For me, I knew that my habit of having a couple of large glasses of wine after a hard day wasn't serving me. I'd carry on working for an hour while I had my first glass, then I'd have another, and by the time it came to eat I thought I might as well have another one with dinner.

I absolutely knew that wasn't helping me towards my weight loss goals and what I wanted to achieve. We probably do know what the problem is and where we could make changes that have a big impact on our results. We just need to take action on it.

## Sustainability

Most people tell me they want sustainability, not just quick weight loss. Things are always going to go wrong at some point. When they do, it's not a failure, as long as you learn for next time. It's not about saying, "this week I didn't get to the gym four times. I can't do this". Instead ask, what did you learn about why you didn't get to the gym four times? Was it because you hadn't planned it in? Was it really a failure if you only got there three times? Start looking at these 'failures' and taking what you can learn for the future.

Many of my clients have a view of failure in the early weeks of the programme. But when we look at the goals they've set, and the weight loss achieved, they realise they haven't failed at all. It is by looking at why they didn't hit their goals and then tweaking it, so they do hit them more regularly and consistently that we succeed.

Consistency leads to habits. Once you have built habits, you get sustainability. Consistency and commitment will create the habit, and the habits will create the sustainability. I drink four litres of water a day. I go to the gym or exercise five times a week. I don't think about it particularly, it just happens out of habit. It couldn't be more sustainable if I wanted it to be. It's effortless. Not because I'm special - I just built the right habits.

You might have to do things, or not do things, to lose weight that you don't want to do forever. Which is fine, making change can require a sacrifice. As my Mum used to say, "We all have to do things we don't want to darling!" Then you must find what you can do forever. The reason people put weight back on is because they stop doing the things that they've learnt, or the things that helped them to lose weight. You must find the things that you enjoy doing. What will you enjoy doing in three weeks' time? What will you enjoy doing in three months' time? What will you enjoy doing in three years' time?

If you don't like weight lifting, don't start by doing weight lifting. If you like the Davina DVD you got for Christmas a year ago, do that. Do the thing that you're going to like doing, to get you into that routine. If you don't like broccoli, don't eat broccoli. If you like green beans, eat green beans. If you don't like eating dry chicken, then put some herbs and spices on it. Make it tasty so you like it.

There's no point in doing stuff that you don't like to lose weight, because you won't sustain it. You must be finding and doing things that you like. That way you carry on doing it, and then it's sustainable.

## Self-Sabotage

Why do we always want to start a diet on another day? After Easter, after Christmas, after our birthday, on Monday, etc. We always say, "I'll start another day". That is just a fear of failure. I think self-sabotage comes in when it gets tough and we think, "I can't do this, so I won't do anything".

Often, we'll make some progress and then we become comfortable. We're a lot better off than we were and we become comfortable in our new zone. Even though we haven't reached our ultimate goal, we feel much better where we are compared to where we began, and we allow ourselves to stop trying. Perhaps we think it's going to be harder to keep progressing. It might not be harder, it might just be different.

There's a big fear of failure that one slip up, a single night out, a single drink, will prove that we can't do this. All we are doing is reinforcing our belief that we can't do it, so we won't try any more. We slip back to the excuses of just being big boned, or menopausal, etc.

It's not the mistakes you make which count, it is what you learn from them. Even if you do just one small thing today that will help you on your journey, it will make a difference. It might just be going out for a walk, turning down the biscuit with your cup of tea in the afternoon, even just being kind to yourself. A lot of people, especially women, are very harsh with themselves about how they look and feel.

I remember once in an exercise class calling myself 'a demented rhino'. The instructor - who's now actually a good friend of mine - asked me why I would say that about myself. Everyone laughed along with me, but the truth was I felt uncomfortable that I couldn't do the exercise, I was embarrassed. It was easier to make a joke than to admit that. If someone else had said that about me, I wouldn't accept it. But it was 'ok' for me to say it to myself.

It's not. It's not ok to talk to yourself like that. You want to try instead to say something positive about yourself. You can learn and reinforce positive behaviours by taking a little bit of time to practice them. Practice being kind to yourself, and positively encouraging yourself, the same way you would a friend or someone else.

## You Can Be Inside-Out Confident

Many people tell me, "oh yes, I'm very confident". Then they hesitate. They aren't inside-out confident, as I call it. A lot of women in my profession, or a lot of women who are professionals in general, are outwardly confident but not inside-out confident. There's a difference. Interestingly, I have also found this with my male clients, that they believe they are judged on how the look, or perceive that they are.

I was outwardly very confident, but inside I was wondering if people think, "yeah she's quite good, but she's a bit tubby". I had this inward lack of belief, but I would still say I was a confident person. I was a competent person, but the inside bit of me hadn't caught up with the outside bit of me.

I'd always wear trousers. I wouldn't wear skirts or dresses, and I don't mean this in the sense of power dressing. It was always trouser suits. I'd never get a skirt suit, and that was simply because I had self-doubt around my body image. Everyone else would say to me, "you always do whatever you set out to achieve". People said that to me, but I didn't believe that I could achieve some of the things I did. Every time I took on a new contract, there would be a sense of, "oh God, am I going to be able to do this? What if I fail?".

When I didn't work for a while, after my Mum died, and then I'd gone into fitness, and I came back out of it, and went back into being an interim again, the voice in the back of my head was asking, "what if I never get a contract? What if I never get another job?".

I'd have these nagging doubts, but when I got to the office, I'd be very competent. Even though sometimes, I wouldn't know what was going on. I remember on one new job, throughout this whole meeting, I had no clue what they were talking about. No clue until someone said to me, "are you alright? You've gone very quiet. Are you keeping up alright?", and I said, "no, not really. I'm a bit confused".

I said, "I know what a GUI is, but what is a guiz?" She said, "Guiz is a person". Ok, of course it's a person. It would always take me quite a long time in myself, to believe I was alright and that I could do it. Outwardly, though, you would never have known that. I knew how to project confidence a lot better than how to feel it.

## Build Confidence By Tracking Your Progress

It's always great to be able to look back on how far you've come. A lot of people put too much focus on the scales. The scales are only one way to track your results and measure what's happening. Remember, what gets measured gets managed. That's why I take measurements and photos with all my clients to ensure we have an accurate picture of what is going on.

People hate the photos to begin with, but when they look back on them they're like, "oh my God! I'm so glad we took these". Knowing you've lost twenty pounds is one thing but seeing it side by side in two photos makes it real. That creates huge levels of confidence when you physically see that transformation. The scales can kill confidence when they don't move, or you at least feel you're doing something wrong. You might be doing everything right and there are other circumstances at play.

There are other ways to track things and you should use a couple of different measurements. This will allow you to get an accurate picture of exactly what is going on, and lead to you building your confidence up as you see results.

I used to do my journal every Thursday on the train on the way home, and I would do a checklist of the things I've done in the week. "I did this, and that, I haven't done this, I haven't done that". Overall, how did I do this week? When you start seeing things that you have done well, you can start to do more of them. Seeing where you struggled, you can make changes to overcome those struggles. Awareness is the key.

Many of the interims I talk to wonder if they are judged on their appearance or whether they're solely judged on their skills and ability. Here's the thing, whether its real or perceived you'll never know, but one of my clients told me, "they told me I wasn't a good cultural fit". She pondered "I wondered if I had the wrong, suit, blouse, necklace or whether I just looked too mumsy".

What is definitely real, is that there's research that shows you are judged on your appearance, even if you're the only one thinking it, of course it could impact your confidence in an interview.

One client said, "I wasn't fulfilling my potential at work. I wasn't speaking up. Then I went to my boss and said, I think I should be managing the new hire. I need to be doing that". She spoke up and did it, and it improved both her own career, and the efficiency of the entire team.

One of my clients decided to take the time to work out of their home environment. By making this decision to work elsewhere, a random email lead to a new opportunity, simply because they were close to the opportunity and went to a meeting that wouldn't have been possible if they were at home.

It depends on what you want to do, but I regularly see this overlap. When you start to get traction in one area of your life, and apply a methodology, you can start to apply it in other areas of your life to do the things that you want to do. Look at me, I gave up my job of over fifteen years, which I was good at and paid well, to get into body transformation coaching and now you're reading my book.

I hadn't really liked being an interim for a long time, but I went back to it after taking time away because it was easy. It was comfortable. I knew that once I got my foot back in the door, once I've got a job, I'll be back to where I was before. Getting that first job was a bit of a challenge because people wondered what I'd been doing the last couple of years. Of course, I was very successful. I could go back to it now, and be very successful doing it, but I didn't like doing it. It didn't make me happy. It wasn't what I wanted to do, and I always knew I wanted to do coaching in some capacity. Then it just got to a certain point and I thought, you've just got to put your money where your mouth is.

*What's the worst that can happen?*

The worst that could happen is I'd have to go back to interim work, if I didn't make a living. I was asking myself, why am I doing something that I don't like. I'm fifty-four, life's too short to do the things that you don't really want to do. Why would I continue to do that?

I knew my confidence had got better, and there was that whole thing my husband said to me before. I can now practice what I preach. I can say to people, "this is how you do it". I've been there, and I've done it myself. That confidence allowed me to take the step to doing what I really wanted with my life.

I can help people. I can motivate people. In the summer just after I'd done my first twelve week transformation I put out my story on Facebook and the response was immense. The amount of people saying, "You're an inspiration. It's amazing. You look fantastic. Look at what you've done".

Wow! I was motivating people. Hopefully they think that if Lisa can do it, I can do it too. Particularly all the people that knew me and hadn't seen me for a long time. The people who would be shocked to see the drastic transformation.

One of my clients had known me from a long time ago— she used to be my cleaner. It was weird, she applied for coaching with me. I called her and said, "are you Amanda that used to do cleaning?". She said yes. I said, "you used to clean for me". She couldn't believe it. She didn't recognise me but when she knew, I think there was that identification, people think, particularly people that used to know me, "if Lisa can do it, I know what Lisa used to be like. Then I can do it too".

It made me feel brilliant. It's so positive. It's that kind of thing that makes you feel amazing, that people would support you in that way, believe in you and start to think, "maybe I can do it too". I believe in you; anything is possible.

People that I don't even know say to me, "you're an inspiration". I had a message from some bloke the other day asking me to connect on LinkedIn, saying, "I've just gone through your story and you were inspirational". A woman messaged me last night, we're connected on Facebook. She said, "I just saw your picture, I thought you looked amazing". If that helps one person to say, "maybe I can do it too", I am so proud. There's always hope for people to make changes in their life.

When you create these values in your physical transformation, you can apply them to other areas of your life. When you create these habits, you can apply them elsewhere. Accepting yourself as who you are today is part of that journey, because who you are today won't be the same person you are tomorrow, or the day after, or in six years' time.

It's not about beating yourself up and being negative, there are too many other people in the world who want to do that. It's just asking, "who I am today?", and loving yourself. It might be a bit difficult, but accepting it is important to moving forwards. Then you can look at who you want to be tomorrow.

We've talked quite a lot about easy wins. Pick out the easy wins, the things that you can do easily to build your confidence. Maybe that's applied even at work. The easy win at work might be, "I'm just going to have a conversation with my peers about different things that we might be able to do to improve". It doesn't necessarily mean going to the boss and saying, "give me a pay rise and a promotion". That could be too big of a step.

The same principles we apply to your physical transformation are applicable in every part of your life. That is where the real value of losing weight comes in. The skills, behaviours, confidence, and habits that you learn can change your life in every area. And on that message, I want to end this book, thank you for reading.

# 8 CONCLUSION

Don't be fooled into thinking you have to make weight loss complicated. People are surprised that it's much easier than they imagined. This plan is for you if you've ever done a diet where you try to change everything, which becomes overwhelming and as soon as something happens outside of the plan, you feel like you've failed.

Making simple changes can bring great success. Two- three changes each week adds up to a lot of change over time. Quite simply, the first thing you can do is be aware of what you're eating by taking photos of your meals. A lot of my clients tell me this really raises the awareness of what they're eating. It's not about being judgmental, just be aware of what you're eating. The next simple change can be to check how much water you're drinking. Then aim to drink a little bit more.

There are two key things you need to remember about diet. One, that it is a simple mathematical equation of calories in versus calories out. To lose weight you need to be in a calorie deficit. The second thing you need to know is that not all calories are created equally. For an average woman, an average number of calories to maintain their weight is 2,000 calories per day. For men it's 2,500. To lose one pound per week you must be in a calorie deficit of 500 calories per day. The second thing is you should focus on eating a good source of protein at every meal. Protein is a super food!

That's a simple rule of thumb, but you don't have to start counting calories straight away. You can do things like reduce your portion sizes or make some swaps for lower calorie foods. Ultimately, you do need to be aware of the number of calories you are eating.

You want to be getting food from high quality sources. I talk about 'single ingredient foods'. That doesn't mean you can't eat some of the things you want, but 80% of the time you want to be using nutrient dense sources of food, rather than calorie dense.

Protein is the key food type. If you increase protein; carbohydrates and fats will take care of themselves. Follow the principle 'what gets measured gets managed' by using My Fitness Pal to gather data and understand where you are. You can download My Fitness Pal app for free to track your food. Remember, it's not about being perfect. It's being in a position where you are in a calorie deficit 80% of the time. Then 20% of the time you can eat some of the things you like to eat.

People often think that exercise is the only thing they need to concentrate on to lose weight, but that is just not the case. Exercise is about 20% of your weight loss efforts. I tell people to think of it as a sweet bonus for weight loss. Of course, it has lots of benefits, but many of these are things you can't see. It's good for heart health, blood pressure, cholesterol levels, etc. But remember, you can't out exercise a bad diet

Whilst you may be able to lose weight on diet alone, if you want to have a nice toned look, you need to exercise to shape your body. Exercise comes in many different forms. The 'best' thing to do is start with whatever you will be consistent and committed with. Find something that you love to do. If you love doing Zumba or a Davina DVD, they are a great place to start.

It is definitely possible to get results with just twenty minutes, three times per week. You don't have to spend hours and hours on the treadmill, or in the gym. The key thing is to start with what you love and build on something that you are going to carry on doing regularly.

Schedule exercise in your diary so you are making that commitment to yourself to do it consistently.

The thing that popular diets don't do is look at your lifestyle. While we are all the same in how we lose weight, they don't account for working a sixty-hour week or commuting ninety minutes each way. It's important to consider your lifestyle and how you manage things. This doesn't have to be complicated. It just takes a little bit of a thought process and planning.

Lots of people say, "I can manage my professional career very well, but I can't seem to manage this". If you apply the same principles you would to a project plan, you break it down and move forwards doing the things that you can do, schedule things in; you create the bandwidth you need to get the results you want.

The main things to do are prioritise the big rocks. Most people know their pinch points. Saying things like, "I'm just so busy that I rush into the nearest place at lunch and grab a sandwich". If you know what your big rocks are, that's the place you can start to create changes.

It's not selfish to take care of yourself. You want to live as long as you possibly can with good health. It's not selfish to want to succeed. It's not selfish to want to take care of yourself. It's not selfish to say "no" to things.

It's ok to not be perfect. If you've got twenty-one meals in the week and five you can't control, you can still succeed if you take care of the other sixteen.

The more you do, the easier this becomes. Don't wait for things to happen, just start doing it. When you take action, other things follow, motivation increases, and it becomes easier. Taking action is the first step to better health and weight loss

It really doesn't matter how old you are. Many people are concerned that they can't lose weight because they're in their forties or fifties; or they have long-term health conditions that could impact their ability to lose weight.

I was at my leanest at age fifty-three. Perhaps it made it harder, but it is definitely possible. I still got in to my best shape ever. Don't think that there's no hope or it's impossible because you're menopausal or peri-menopausal. It might take longer to reach your goal, but it is always possible. Trust the process and give it a go; you will see results.

We all have periods in our life where things overtake us. It's difficult to stick with the routine sometimes, when you've had a bad day, you're stressed, etc. Having a glass of wine or not giving attention to what you are eating in the short term doesn't really matter, but if it's something that you must deal with on a regular basis, it will impact your weight loss.

If you don't manage stress you will struggle with weight loss. It's important you deal with it in the best possible way you can. Firstly, identify what the stress triggers in your life are, and what your coping mechanisms are. Then you can look at if you could do something differently. Second, simply accept it. Go with the flow and make sure you treat yourself kindly, get plenty of rest and sleep.

Motivation is an interesting topic. People say to me, "I just need to get motivated". If I had a quid every time someone said that to me, I'd be very rich. Motivation will get you started, but it won't take you to your goal. The reality is, if you take action you gain confidence, and with confidence comes motivation. It's the other way around to what many people assume.

You don't need to be motivated to drink more water or eat five portions of vegetables a day, you can just start doing it. Have faith that if you take action, you will become more confident and more motivated.

The aesthetics of losing weight will take you so far, but it won't keep you going in the long term. Take a pen and paper and write down every reason why it's important for you to lose weight. Is it about being around for your children? Worries about your health? Is it impacting your confidence getting jobs and costing you money?

As your mindset starts to change and you see progress, you will begin creating new habits. You'll know that simple changes create results, so you can build them as habits, which are essential to long term success. It's not like a diet that has a beginning and an end. Its making small switches that become routine and form new habits.

You need to make a commitment to yourself. Set specific goals and write them down. Don't just say, "I'm going to lose two pounds". When I work with my clients I'm asking them how are they going to lose two pounds? Be very clear and specific in your action steps.

Remember that progress is not just about the number on the scales. Tracking by taking pictures of yourself and taking your measurements are important metrics to see your progress and build confidence.

We often sabotage ourselves on diets because we feel restricted, get off track and then think we have failed. Or we have a 'friendly saboteur'— a well-meaning friend or family member who is encouraging us to fall off track. Another way we sabotage ourselves is failing to make an appropriate plan.

It's important to recognise that there is no such thing as failure. You don't have to restrict yourself. Just because you eat something doesn't mean you have failed. If you want to have something, have it and enjoy it. Just admit why you're having it and recognise how it will impact your goals.

Building your confidence is key. One of my clients lost sixteen pounds in twelve weeks, but she was down three dress sizes. Would you be happy losing three dress sizes? It's not just about focusing on the scales. When you track and see progress your confidence will increase.

You can take these principles and use them in other parts of your life to increase your confidence. Such as working on two- three small changes. Many people tell me that when they start losing weight it spills over into improvement in many other areas of their life. You can achieve other goals with the same techniques.

If there's one thing that I can stress more than anything it is that small changes, the simplicity of breaking it down to bite-sized chunks can lead to major results. Do that consistently, with commitment and you will succeed. Don't see this as a punishment, enjoy the journey along the way, and remember if you focus on the inputs, the outcome will take care of itself.

# 9 NEXT STEPS

As I've mentioned throughout this book, the most important thing to do is to take action.

When I cleared my house to move to Spain, I found about twenty diet books— this is after I had cleared my house to move from London to Hastings and thrown out about 30 of them!

I don't know why I had so many. As one of my clients said to me, "I've got every diet book going"…

So I get it, *Project You* could just be another 'diet' book, sitting gathering dust on your bookshelf as you think, "Yeah, that's quite interesting, I'll give it a go some time".

But, maybe you read something that struck a chord. Maybe you read about one of my awesome clients and thought, "That sounds just like me, if she can do it, why not me".

You may realise that now is the time to work on fixing your weight problem once and for all. That accountability, support and the help to implement a simple "no diet formula" plan tailored to your situation is what you need.

I am grateful that you've bought my book and taken the time to read this far. If you want to take the next step to success and find out more about my 12 Week Project You transformation programme, please email me Lisa@LisaAliCoach.com and quote "BOOK" for a special BONUS worth

$199— "Gym in a bag" — the only two pieces of kit you need, which you can take anywhere from home to hotel to get a super effective workout with the best fat burning exercises.

Believe me when I say there is always hope and you can do it. Find out more at www.LisaAliCoach.com.

# ABOUT THE AUTHOR

Lisa Ali is a Body Transformation Coach who loves to help interim managers and consultants to achieve weight loss and be their most happy, healthy, confident selves. More importantly, Lisa was an interim manager for many years and understands the challenges of the lifestyle, stress and demands that often go hand in hand with contract work.
She has over five years' experience in the health and fitness industry, and finally found the formula to successful weight loss, even when working a ten plus hour day and undergoing her own personal body transformation losing a total of forty-five pounds.

She has now shared this formula with other busy professionals to help them transform their bodies and lives. Her work has been featured in the Daily Mail and she is a regular contributor to Talk Radio Europe.

You can connect with her at www.lisaalicoach.com

Printed in Great Britain
by Amazon